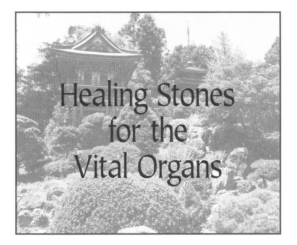

Healing Stones
for the
Vital Organs

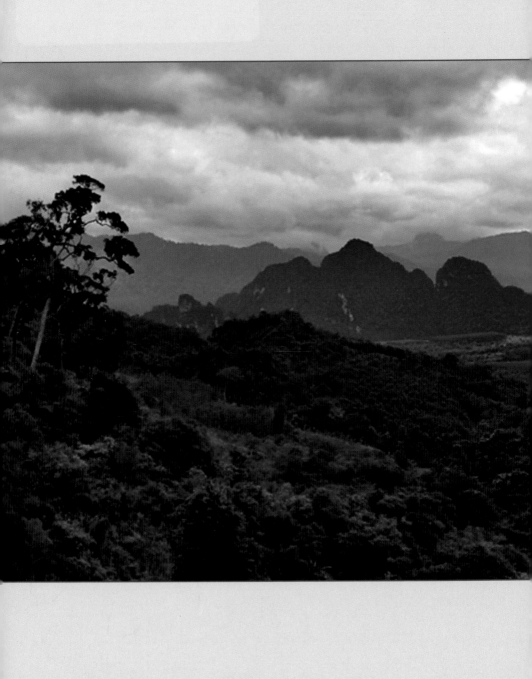

Healing Stones
for the
Vital Organs

◆

83 Crystals with
Traditional Chinese Medicine

Michael Gienger and Wolfgang Maier

Translated by Ariel Godwin

Healing Arts Press

Rochester, Vermont

Healing Arts Press
One Park Street
Rochester, Vermont 05767
www.HealingArtsPress.com

Healing Arts Press is a division of Inner Traditions International

Originally published in German under the title *Heilsteine der Organuhr* by Neue
Erde
First U.S. edition published in 2009 by Healing Arts Press

Note to the reader: *This book is intended as an informational guide. The remedies,
approaches, and techniques described herein are meant to supplement, and not to be a
substitute for, professional medical care or treatment. They should not be used to treat
a serious ailment without prior consultation with a qualified health care professional.*

Library of Congress Cataloging-in-Publication Data
Gienger, Michael.
 [Heilsteine der Organuhr. English]
 Healing stones for the vital organs : 83 crystals with traditional Chinese medicine
/ Michael Gienger and Wolfgang Maier ; translated from the German by Ariel
Godwin. —1st U.S. ed.
  p. cm.
 Includes bibliographical references and index.
 ISBN 978-1-59477-275-7 (pbk.)
 1. Precious stones—Therapeutic use. 2. Crystals—Therapeutic use. 3. Medicine,
Chinese. I. Maier, Wolfgang. II. Title.
 RZ560.G54 2009
 615.8'52—dc22

                                                              2008048854

Printed and bound in India by Replika Press Pvt. Ltd.

10 9 8 7 6 5 4 3 2 1

Text design and layout by Virginia Scott Bowman
This book was typeset in Garamond Premier Pro and Futura with Tiepolo, Futura,
and Gil Sans as display typefaces

Contents

———————◆———————

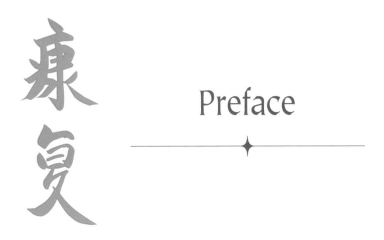

Preface

THE ORGAN CLOCK in traditional Chinese medicine is a magnificent aid for the early identification of energy disturbances that, in the long run, can lead to bodily illness or psychic ailments. With the organ clock, the specific conditions of illness can be recognized and swiftly remedied. It is an instrument for the maintenance of health, applicable to both prevention and treatment of disease.

For these reasons, the organ clock has been used for diagnosis and therapy since the beginning of modern crystal healing. Its clear structure and ease of manipulation make it a useful aid for laypeople as well, for self-healing and preventive maintenance. Hardly any other medicinal system is so simple in its practical application.

The challenge in coordinating the connection between healing stones and the organ clock has been in identifying the appropriate healing stones for the resolution of specific energy disturbances and in treating the discomfort or illness resulting from those disturbances. Initially, the differing views of Western and Chinese medicine were not easy to reconcile.

The first correspondences of healing stones to the organ clock were very much influenced by Western thought and Western interpretations of the organs and bodily functions. Through practical experimentation, "functional correspondences" emerged, but their effect initially was limited predominantly to symptoms, usually not reaching the level of the actual cause of illness. This was sufficient for use as a home remedy but not for lasting therapeutic application.

Thanks to Wolfgang Maier's more than fifteen years of research, a deeper level of the connection between crystal healing and the organ clock can now be presented. His precise illustration of the twelve function areas of the organ clock, based on yin and yang as well as on the five phases of change, makes it possible to provide a classification of healing stones at the causative level.

The healing stones for the organ clock introduced in this book, therefore, correspond to the energetic seeds of bodily illnesses and psychic disturbances. Their effect is etiological; they allow problems to be identified at their origins and, so to speak, pulled out by the roots. Their therapeutic effect is thus substantially greater and more enduring.

The energetic foundations and correspondences are outlined in this book as simply and understandably as possible. This guide is intended to make the application of healing stones, with the help of the organ clock, available to all who are interested—laypeople and therapists alike. Self-healing is more important today than it once was, and it is for this purpose that the organ clock was originally developed. With this book, we hope to make a small contribution to the health of all beings.

MICHAEL GIENGER
TÜBINGEN, GERMANY

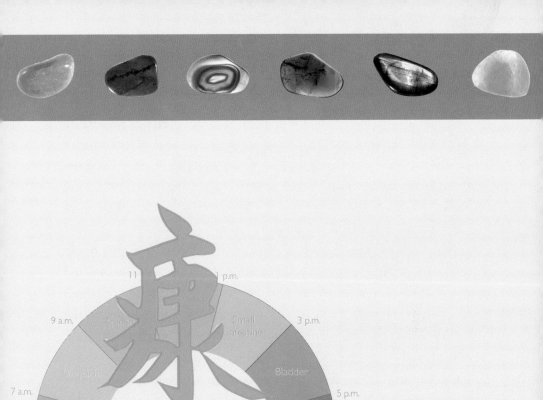

Ancient Tools for
Timely Healing

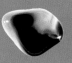

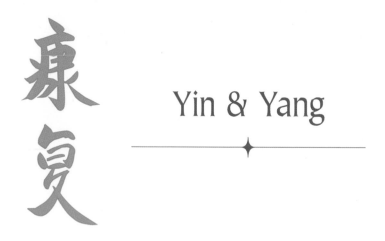

Yin & Yang

ALL OF CHINESE PHILOSOPHY—and consequently all of traditional Chinese medicine—is based on the principles of yin and yang. Static, passive yin and dynamic, active yang are the two laws that together form the basis of all existence, and from which all things originate.

WHAT ARE YIN AND YANG?

Everything that tends outward and upward, all that is active and dynamic, is yang. In contrast, all that tends inward and downward, all that is heavy and substantial, is yin. When we look at the contrast between matter and energy, matter is yin and energy is yang. In comparing day and night, day is yang and night is yin. Yin and yang forever describe the relationship of two opposites to one another.

EVERYTHING IS CHANGING

The idea of yin and yang is an idea of eternal change. Yin changes into yang and yang back into yin. Thus day emerges from night, growing ever brighter, reaching its high point, and finally, inevitably, beginning to wane. Noon, the brightest point of the day, is also the beginning of the day's ending. In other words, when yang (here, brightness) is strongest, yin (here, darkness) begins to increase. Likewise, the summer sol-

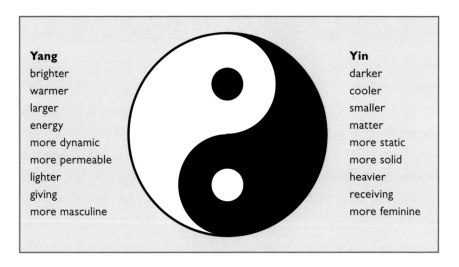

Yang	Yin
brighter	darker
warmer	cooler
larger	smaller
energy	matter
more dynamic	more static
more permeable	more solid
lighter	heavier
giving	receiving
more masculine	more feminine

stice is the high point of the brighter time of the year but is also the beginning of the transition toward the darker time of the year.

ALL THINGS EMERGE FROM OPPOSITES

Just as light is not imaginable without darkness (without either, there would be eternal twilight), so yin cannot exist without yang, and vice versa. The one requires the other, just as the front side of a wall requires its back side. A wall with only one side simply cannot exist.

YIN AND YANG ARE RELATIVE

Mountains are larger than people. Thus a mountain is yang in relation to a person, and a person is yin in relation to a mountain. People are larger than flies. Thus a person is yang in relation to a fly, and a fly is yin in relation to a person.

So is a person yin or yang?

A fire is yang in relation to a cold pile of logs but yin in relation to the sun. Yin and yang are always connected to the relationship between two things. So the saying that yin is darkness and yang is light, that heat is yang and cold is yin, is correct yet imprecise.

Yin is darker than yang; yang is lighter than yin.

EXTREMES CHANGE
INTO THEIR OPPOSITES

There is no absolute darkness, because darkness changes back into light.

There is no limitless heat, for cooling always must follow eventually.

There is no eternal height; after reaching the highest point, a descent must follow.

Yang, at its maximum, changes into yin; and yin, at its extreme, becomes yang.

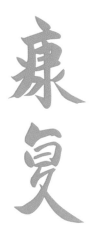

The Five Phases
of Change

IN CHINA, MILLENNIA OF OBSERVATIONS in nature gave rise to the system of the "five phases of change." Each phase of change corresponds to a specific element for which it is named. All processes in life and in nature go through five steps: beginning, expansion, high point, retreat, and end (completion). The five phases of change reflect this principle: The phase of water is the beginning of everything. Expansion takes place in the phase of wood, reaching the high point in the phase of fire. Metal is the phase of retreat, and at the end of everything there is water again. The fifth phase, the phase of earth, is usually placed between fire and metal. This is the phase of duration, the time when things are steady and lasting in the world; the phase of beingness. The harmony of this cycle is the basis for health in humans. Disturbances and disharmony lead to illness.

The phases of change describe the progression of the seasons and the passage of the day on the organ clock. They explain the interplay of the twelve function areas of the clock and indicate which influences lead to illness or preserve health. Whereas Western medicine recognizes and addresses only the physical (in this case, specific internal organs), treatment of the function areas embraces organs and bodily structures as well as the senses, emotions, psychic aspects, and spiritual capabilities connected with them.

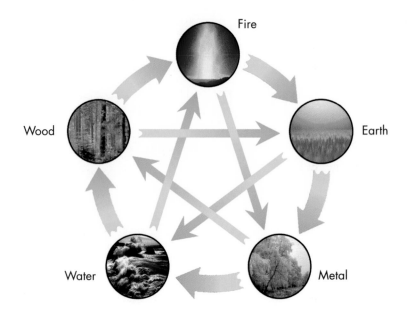

WOOD

The change phase of wood is the phase of construction and growth. The primary qualities of wood are *flexibility* and *creativity;* flexibility for adapting to external conditions, and creativity for surmounting obstacles and creating optimal situations. Assertiveness, required in order to gain and maintain a place in life, also belongs to wood; likewise the sinews and muscles that serve for movement, and the fingernails and toenails that serve as rudimentary claws. The season of wood is spring, the time of growth and beginnings. The change phase of wood corresponds to the function areas of the liver and gallbladder.

FIRE

The change phase of fire is pure *action, exuberance,* and the *zest for life,* movement out of joy and enthusiasm for "being in the moment." Fire is warmth and light. It is vibrant and energizing, active, brilliant, exciting, and colorful. Fire corresponds to the season of summer, the time of year for the greatest amount of activity. Spirit belongs to fire, corresponding to our true nature. As a vocal expression, laughter, a sign of joy in life, corresponds to fire. The function areas of fire are the heart, small intestine, pericardium, and triple heater.

EARTH

The change phase of earth is the center and source of all the other phases of change. Every life, every condition, all that is material emerges from earth, has its roots in earth, grows from earth, and returns to it upon death. To be "grounded" means to be balanced and consistent in the play of forces in the world. The change phase of earth rules the *rhythmic forces* in nature and in our bodies—it governs the changing of the seasons and natural changes in nature. The season of the change phase of earth is late summer, the time of ripening and harvest. The nature of earth corresponds most to the ample wealth of the present day, in which food is plentiful. Earth does not correspond to any direction; it is the center. Its function areas are the spleen and stomach.

METAL

The change phase of metal represents *firmness* and *stability*. Metal holds things together, binds them and makes exchange possible. Thus communication and contact, the interplay between being too close and being too far, also belong to metal. The vocal expression of metal is crying, which happens when connections are broken or when a desired connection is denied. The season of metal is autumn, the time of transition and letting go. The skin, the greatest contact organ of the body, corresponds to metal, as do the function areas of the lungs and large intestine, which are responsible for assimilating and eliminating.

WATER

We are water! Inside the human body there are reservoirs, rivers, seas, oceans of energy, springs of life. Water is the source of inner *movement* and *adaptability*. Water is the origin of the ability to act and the strength of will, and therefore of the ability to reach goals. The actual capacity to act, however, is not a part of water but of the change phases of wood and fire. The bones, whose stability and strength carry the body, are expressions of the change phase of water. It is the reservoir of life energy and is full of potential. The season of water is winter, when the world rests and rebuilds its energy to use in the coming year. The function areas of the kidneys and bladder correspond to water.

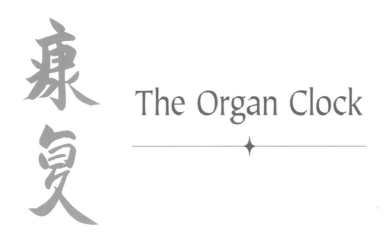

The Organic Clock

FUNCTION AREAS AND ORGANS

The twelve function areas in traditional Chinese medicine are mostly named after specific organs. They are not organs as delineated by Western medicine but instead represent a much broader concept, embracing multilevel bodily functions, emotions, psychic aspects, and spiritual abilities.

The term *organ clock,* however, has become established in the literature, and therefore it is used in this text.

EXCHANGE BETWEEN ACTIVITY AND REST

The twelve function areas are not equally active and productive at any given time; rather, they have individual high and low phases throughout the course of the day. These phases occur in a fixed rhythm corresponding to the path of the sun. A function area is especially active at the time of day best suited for the performance of its duties.

The activity of a function area does not decrease abruptly but in a gently descending curve, reaching its low point after twelve hours, then rising again from there.

ONE AFTER THE OTHER

Each function area works with its greatest strength for two hours daily. As soon as its activity wanes, the next function area reaches its own

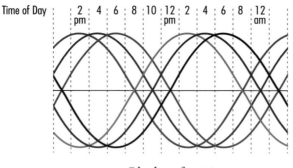

Rhythm of activity

high point of activity. Thus the high points of the function areas alternate in a two-hour rhythm. The organ clock shows the rhythmic progression of these high points. The function area indicated for a specific time of day reaches its maximum activity during this time. At the same time, the function area on the opposite side of the organ clock is at its low point of activity, while the other areas are at different degrees of strength and weakness.

THE SUN'S PATH

The high points of activity in the function areas are aligned with the sun. "Noon" on the organ clock is the time when the sun is at its highest point. Since this differs depending on latitude, "real time" must generally be calculated for the use of the organ clock. How this works is explained in the chapter Calculating Real Local Time.

HELP FROM THE ORGAN CLOCK

With the help of the organ clock, disturbances in the function areas can be recognized early on and treated, often long before they lead to illness. Someone who often awakens between 1:00 and 3:00 in the morning probably has a disturbance in the function area of the liver. Someone who feels very tired around 2:00 p.m. may have problems with small intestine function. As soon as such things are identified, the problems can be tackled. (This will be discussed in the following chapter, Application of Healing Stones.)

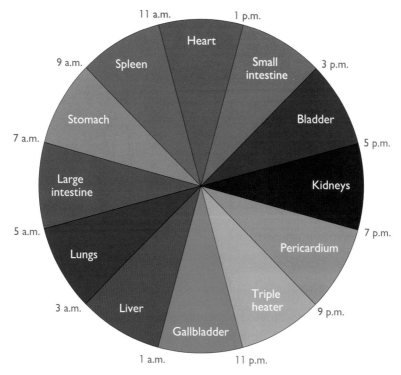

The organ clock

It is important to remember that the times of day given here refer to real local time, which can differ from standard time. (See Calculating Real Local Time, beginning on page 24.)

PREVENTION WITH THE ORGAN CLOCK

"Prevention is better than healing," so the saying goes. This is especially true in Chinese medicine; this principle was observed so consistently in ancient China that doctors were paid only when their patients stayed healthy.

The organ clock allows easy discernment of which activities are best suited to which time of day, and which should be avoided, if possible, because they lead to overstraining and thus, over the long term, to illness. Synchronizing your daily life with the organ clock may seem difficult at first but is a very effective way to preserve good health to a ripe old age.

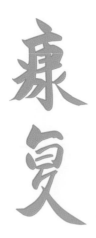

Application of Healing Stones

HEALING STONES CAN BE APPLIED in many different ways for balancing out disturbances in the function areas and thus preventing or healing illnesses.

CHOOSING THE RIGHT STONES

Every application begins with choosing the right stones. For this, study the chapter, The Five Phases of Change, and those chapters within the second part of the book, Function Areas: Physical and Psychic Aspects of Healing, first checking the descriptions of the individual healing stones for each function area in order to get an overview. In doing this, take notes on the themes related to each function area.

Now look over your notes and decide which theme is most important at the moment. If this decision is difficult, do it by elimination, progressively eliminating the less important themes until you have isolated the central theme.

This should at least bring you to the point of focusing on a single function area. If several different themes within this function area stand out to you, this is normal. But in order to choose the right healing stone, it is also important to look within the function area and see which theme interests you most, then proceed with it.

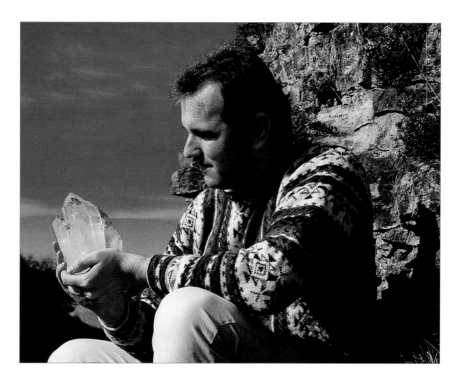

Once you have found or chosen a central theme, read the descriptions of the corresponding healing stones and decide which stone fits best. If this is a difficult decision, select as small a number as possible of appealing healing stones and compare their descriptions with those in the other themes of the function area.

The healing stone with the overall description that fits you best is the right stone for you.

If you still feel uncertain, discuss the choice of your stone with someone you trust. The spectator can often see more of the game than the players, and can help clarify the right choice. You can also check your choices by searching in other books. For this, Michael Gienger's *Healing Crystals: The A–Z Guide to 430 Gemstones* is especially recommended.* You can also consult professional healing stone advisers and therapists.

---

*Publication information for this and other recommended books are provided in the Recommended Reading section. (See page 169.)

Summary: Choosing the Right Healing Stones

✦ Study the text and note the applicable themes.

✦ Identify the most important function areas.

✦ Choose the most relevant themes within the function area.

✦ Decide on the most appropriate healing stone.

If you are familiar with processes of energy testing (dowsing, kinesiology, and so on), you can use them to test your choice of healing stone and to establish the proper point in time and duration for application (see the following sections).

USING THE ORGAN CLOCK

The organ clock itself can give direct advice as to which function areas have a causal involvement in certain complaints or illnesses. The times at which certain disturbances arise or intensify are directly connected to the times of the function areas given in the organ clock.

Disturbances caused by excessive functioning often emerge precisely at the function area's peak time, as shown on the organ clock (see page 11).

Disturbances caused by suppressed function often manifest during the lowest time of the function area in question, twelve hours before and after its peak time (and thus at the exact opposite point on the organ clock).

It is very important to note that here we are referring to "real time," which may differ from "standard time" (see page 24).

Thus, waking up regularly at 4:00 a.m. may indicate excessive lung function (this being the peak time of the lungs), or else a weak bladder (being the bladder's lowest point). Symptoms will often indicate which function area is causing the problem: if waking up coughing and wheezing as an effect of smoking cigarettes, the lungs are endeavoring to forcefully clear themselves. But awakening completely exhausted yet desperately needing to urinate is much more likely to indicate bladder weakness.

Hyperactive energy, hot flushes, pain, tension, and bloated feelings are especially strong indicators of excessive functioning; whichever function area is currently nearest its peak time is most likely the one to blame.

Lack of energy, weakness, malfunctioning, chills, and sensory disturbances are indicators of suppressed function, in whichever function area is nearest its low point at the time of the symptoms.

However, these indications are only approximate. The symptoms of excessive and deficient function are covered more thoroughly in the following delineation of the twelve function areas. With the help of these descriptions, it will be easier to ascertain which function area is affected by a disturbance.

In any case, the organ clock helps to identify which function area is affected by a disturbance by allowing us to observe precisely when symptoms emerge, worsen, or diminish. These observations should always be taken into consideration in the choice of healing stones.

Summary: Using the Organ Clock

✦ The time at which symptoms occur or intensify generally coincides with the highest or lowest point of the function area in question.

✦ This means that the function area occupying this time (peak time) or the one lying directly opposite (lowest time) is likely the one affected.

✦ The symptoms themselves often suggest a conclusion regarding which function area is affected (if necessary, compare the descriptions of the twelve function areas).

✦ Excessive functions are often expressed at the peak time by a surplus of energy, heat flushes, pain, tension, or "full" feelings.

✦ Suppressed functions are often expressed at the lowest time by a lack of energy, weakness, malfunctioning, chills, and sensory disturbances.

✦ The direct indications of the organ clock should always be taken into account in the choice of healing stones.

TIME AND DURATION

The duration of treatment and the choice of the right point in time play an important role in the use of healing stones. At the beginning of treatment with a newly chosen healing stone, it is sometimes best to apply it as often as possible, even around the clock. If the need is present, it certainly is an option. But if this initially leads to a worsening of certain symptoms prior to improvement (much as in homeopathic medicine, this is often the case with healing stones), there is a choice either to wait it out or switch to a brief course of regular treatment. Naturally, in the case of worsening symptoms or serious illness, a doctor, healer, or therapist should be consulted.

If there is no need to wear the stone constantly, or if this is inadvisable due to a strong increase in symptoms, standard brief treatment is recommended. The organ clock itself indicates the best possible times. As a rule, a function area is most treatable when its levels of energy and activity are rising. This means the peak time suggested by the organ clock, as well as the six hours or so leading up to that time. Healing stones applied during this time for ten to twenty minutes, or worn for between half an hour and two hours, will have an enduring effect on the function area. The nearer to the peak time the better, although practical considerations should always be observed. For example, it is better to treat the liver with healing stones in the evening before going to bed rather than waking up especially to do so at 2:00 a.m. If each treatment is repeated daily at the same time, the effectiveness will be equal, or even superior, to round-the-clock treatment.

With regular brief treatments, an initial worsening of symptoms is rare and usually slight. If this causes discomfort, try reducing the duration of treatment (for example, to five minutes' application or wearing for fifteen minutes), then increasing it each day.

Summary: Time and Duration

✦ Constant application, if desired and comfortable.

✦ Regular brief treatment, if desired, or in the case of a strong initial setback.

✦ Regular brief treatment at, or prior to, the peak time of the function area.

✦ Be practical when choosing times (respecting breaks, sleep, and so on).

✦ Duration of regular treatment: ten to twenty minutes application or half an hour to two hours' wearing.

✦ If symptoms worsen initially, reduce treatment time, then slowly increase it day by day.

When determining times, take into account the fact that the organ clock is always set to sunrise, or "real time" (see page 24).

METHODS OF APPLICATION

Methods of application consist of either local applications or general applications.

⚐ LOCAL APPLICATION

Local applications are mainly appropriate when localized complaints are present. The corresponding healing stone is placed, or fixed, upon

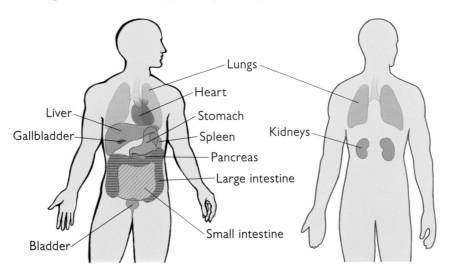

Application areas corresponding to the physical organs

the area of complaint. For affixing the stone, breathable bandage tape, gauze, or similar material should be used.

Another advantage to local applications is that by choosing the point or area to treat, specific function areas can be addressed. This applies to the areas in which the corresponding physical organs are located and to special organ areas on the abdomen and back. The meridian end points on the hands and feet are also possible treatment areas, for example using rings made of stone. (For treatment to be effective the stone must be touching the skin.) For those familiar with acupuncture, acupressure, shiatsu, and traditional Chinese medicine,

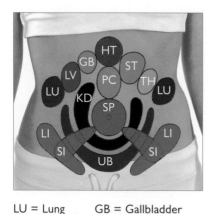
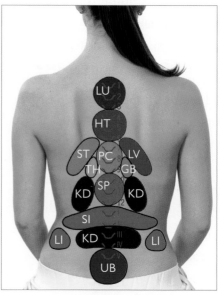

LU = Lung	GB = Gallbladder
LV = Liver	PC = Pericardium
HT = Heart	TH = Triple Heater
ST = Stomach	LI = Large Intestine
KD = Kidney	SI = Small Intestine
SP = Spleen	UB = Urinary Bladder

Organ zones on the abdomen and back

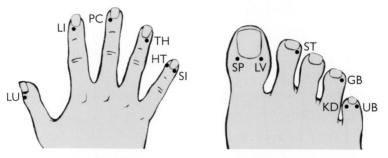

Meridian end points on the hands and feet

the acupuncture points on the meridians can, naturally, also be used.

If you have practiced with healing stones for a long time, follow your instincts or your experience in choosing among these possibilities.

Summary: Local Applications

For local complaints or direct treatment of specific function areas:

✦ Place or affix healing stones on or near the affected area.

For direct treatment of specific function areas, work with the following regions:

✦ The location of the physical organ associated with the function area.
✦ Organ zones on the back and abdomen.
✦ Meridian points on the hands and feet.
✦ Acupuncture points on the meridians (for those familiar with them).

⚔ GENERAL APPLICATION

General applications are particularly appropriate when multiple areas or entire bodily systems need to be treated: blood, circulation, the triple heater, nerves, hormones, and so on; as well as for body-wide ailments such as rheumatism, autoimmune diseases, allergies, and disturbances in metabolism; and for problems that affect body, soul, and spirit simultaneously.

Here, healing stones are worn externally or imbibed as healing stone water or elixir. Healing stone massages also offer wonderful possibilities.

The simplest applications involve wearing healing stones as pendants, collars, or bracelets on the ankles or wrists. A good place for pendants intended to have a general effect on body, soul, and spirit is the area of the thymus, halfway between the heart and larynx. Chains worn around the neck and bracelets worn on the ankles or wrists will reach the blood, lymph, nerves, and meridians that run through these points (six out of the twelve in each case), treating all areas of the body and all aspects of life. The same naturally goes for imbibing healing stone

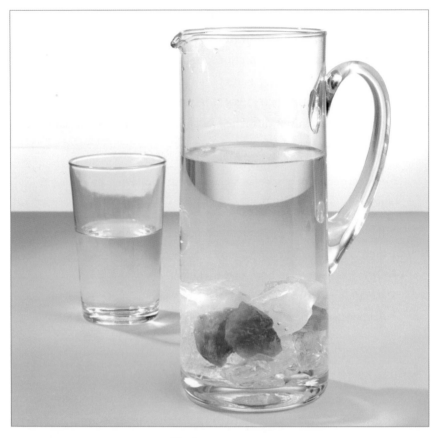

Healing stone water

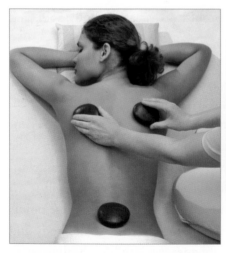

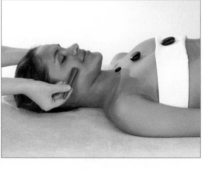

Healing stone massage

water and elixirs, which distribute the stone's information throughout the whole body and energy system. But since these internal medicines must be administered with great care, be sure to educate yourself before trying it: see Michael Gienger and Joachim Goebel, *Gem Water: How to Prepare and Use Over 130 Crystal Waters for Therapeutic Treatments*. For techniques of healing stone massage, see Dagmar Fleck and Liane Jochum, *Hot Stone and Gem Massage* or Michael Gienger's *Crystal Massage for Health and Healing*.

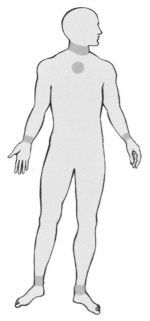

Effective areas for general (full coverage) application

Summary: General Applications

✦ For treating multiple areas, body-wide systems, or body, soul, and spirit simultaneously.

✦ Healing stones can be worn as pendants, collars, or bracelets, especially on the neck, near the thymus, on the wrists, or on the ankles.

✦ Internal consumption of healing stone water and healing stone elixirs is also an option, but great care must be taken.

✦ Healing stone massages are an excellent option for highly effective overall healing.

CLEANSING THE STONES

Before and after use, healing stones must be energetically cleansed in order to flush out energy they have absorbed. Someone else's information stored in a stone could have an undesirable influence on its healing effects.

⚔ DISCHARGING

To discharge a healing stone, hold it under lukewarm running water for at least one minute, rubbing vigorously with the fingers until the soapy feeling is gone from the surface. The stone is then discharged, or freed from excess energy. Stone necklaces or bracelets on string should simply be rubbed with a damp cloth, since immersion might damage the strings. Water-soluble stones, for example rock salt (halite), should not be discharged with water. For these stones, cleanse on the amethyst crystals only (see page 23).

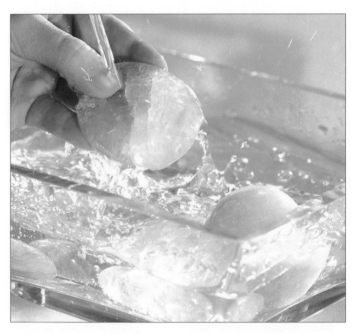

Discharging excess energy

⚔ CLEANSING

Following the discharging, the healing stones (including necklaces and bracelets) should then be left for at least two to three hours on a bed of amethyst crystals. Amethyst releases all kinds of sticky energy and thoroughly frees the healing stones placed on it from all "foreign" information. Afterward, the stones are like new and in the best condition for healing purposes.

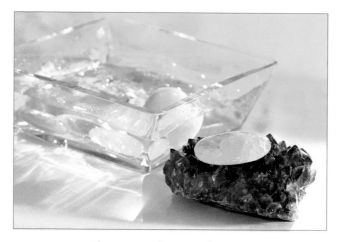

Clearing out foreign information

Placing upon amethyst is recommended for all healing stones except amber. Amber is fossilized resin, and information becomes fixed in amber more tenaciously than in other stones. It is best to discharge it under lukewarm running water and then leave it in full sunlight for several days. This is the only way to remove a significant amount of foreign information from amber.

In addition to these processes, healing stones can also be cleansed with smoke, sound vibrations, and special ceremonies. But discharging under running water followed by purification on amethyst is the necessary minimum procedure that invariably should be followed. For more information on cleansing stones, see Michael Gienger's *Purifying Crystals: How to Clear, Charge and Purify Your Healing Crystals.*

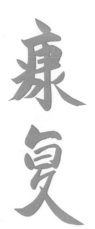

Calculating Real Local Time

THE ORGAN CLOCK IS CONTINUALLY SYNCHRONIZED with the passage of the sun, that is "real local time" rather than "universal time" or "standard time." In real local time it is 6:00 a.m. when the sun is due east; 12:00 noon when it reaches its highest point in the sky; and 6:00 p.m. when it is due west. Consequently, each place has its own local time. In New York's local time, for example, 12:00 noon occurs twenty-four minutes earlier than in Miami.

In the late nineteenth century, local times were generally synchronized and time zones were created. For example, in eastern North America, the same time zone (EST = eastern standard time) reaches from the Atlantic to Lake Superior, even though the sun takes an hour and a half to pass over this whole region. This means that the sun reaches its highest point in the sky over Eastport, Maine at 11:30 a.m. But in Ontonagon, Michigan, it does not reach its highest point until 1:00 p.m. So "local time" and "standard time" can be quite different.

But because our bodies continue to follow the sun, rather than a standard time agreed upon for political convenience, we must take this difference into account when dealing with the organ clock. So, once again, here is the definition of *real time:* When the sun is at its highest point at a given place, from the body's point of view it is noon at this location.

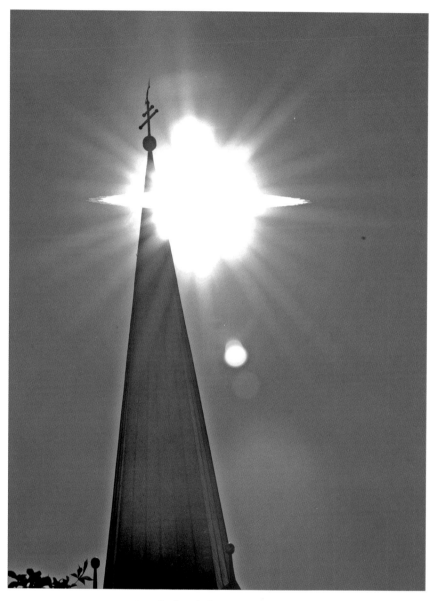

Our bodies define noon *as when
the sun is at its highest point in the sky.*

In order to calculate real time, we must know the location at which real time and standard time are actually the same, then locate our position to the east or west.

For each North American time zone, there is a degree of longitude at which local time coincides with standard time. These lines of longitude are as follows:

- **NST** (Newfoundland standard time): 52.5° west
- **AST** (Atlantic standard time): 60° west
- **EST** (eastern standard time): 75° west
- **CST** (central standard time): 90° west
- **MST** (mountain standard time): 105° west
- **PST** (Pacific standard time): 120° west
- **AKST** (Alaskan standard time): 135° west
- **HAST** (Hawaii-Aleutian standard Time): 150° west

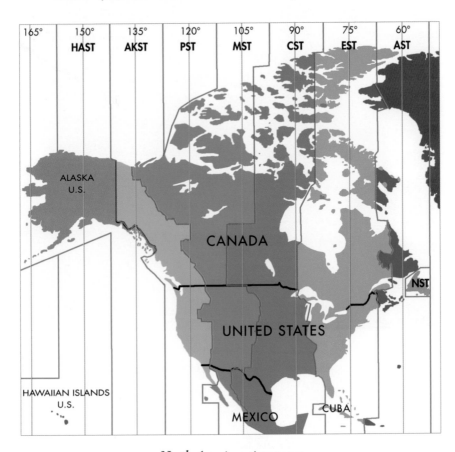

North American time zones

At all locations that fall exactly upon the lines of longitude listed above (and are in the corresponding time zone), standard time is identical to real local time. If a place within a given time zone lies east of that time zone's line of longitude, then the sun reaches its highest point before noon at that location. Therefore, local time is ahead of standard time. At places west of the line of longitude, the sun reaches its highest point after 12:00 noon. Therefore, local time is behind standard time.

East of the given line of longitude, local time is ahead of standard time. West of the line of longitude, local time is behind standard time.

By using an atlas, one can determine the degree to which local time is earlier or later than standard time. The sun takes twenty-four hours to "travel" around the 360° of the earth. Consequently, it takes one hour to travel 15° (360° / 24 = 15°), and four minutes to travel 1° (60 / 15 = 4). In a particular location, for each degree east or west of the line of longitude where local time and standard time are the same, four minutes must be added or subtracted in order to calculate local time.

EXAMPLE FOR A LOCATION IN THE EASTERN TIME ZONE

Local time in the eastern time zone corresponds to the 75th meridian west of Greenwich. If we are to the east of the 75th meridian, we must add four minutes for each degree of difference. If we are west of the 75th meridian, on the other hand, we must subtract four minutes for each degree of difference.

Example: Washington, D.C., lies at 77° west, consequently 2° west of the 75th meridian. In order to calculate local time, we must subtract 2 x 4 = 8 minutes from eastern standard time. When the clocks show 12:00 noon (EST), real local time in Washington, D.C., is 11:52 a.m.

Quebec City, on the other hand, lies at 71° west, which is 4° to the east of the 75th meridian. To calculate local time, we must add 4 x 4 = 16 minutes to eastern standard time. When the clocks show 12:00 noon (EST), local time in Quebec City is 12:16 p.m.

This is the entire "secret" of real time: If we know which meridian corresponds to the intersection of real time and standard time in our time zone, then we can consult an atlas to determine how far we are (in degrees) and in which direction (east or west) from that meridian. Then standard time can be appropriately corrected: going east, add four minutes per degree; going west, subtract four minutes per degree. And that's it!

GREENWICH MEAN TIME

Greenwich mean time (GMT) is used as a basis for the calculation of time worldwide; it corresponds to the meridian of zero degrees, which runs through Greenwich in London. All other time zones worldwide are coordinated to GMT.

For time zones in North America, this means:

NST (Newfoundland standard time): GMT – 3½ hours
AST (Atlantic standard time): = GMT – 4 hours
EST (eastern standard time): = GMT – 5 hours
CST (central standard time): = GMT – 6 hours
MST (mountain standard time): = GMT – 7 hours
PST (Pacific standard time): = GMT – 8 hours
AKST (Alaskan standard time): = GMT – 9 hours
HAST (Hawaii-Aleutian satndard time): = GMT – 10 hours

You can thus proceed worldwide:

If you know the meridian line to which a given time zone corresponds, you can then determine your position east or west of that meridian line, and your distance from it.

Then, as detailed previously, you can calculate your local time as distinct from standard time.

CORRECTING FOR DAYLIGHT SAVING TIME

In summer, an additional factor must be observed, which is not the same in all countries: daylight saving time. Daylight saving time in the United

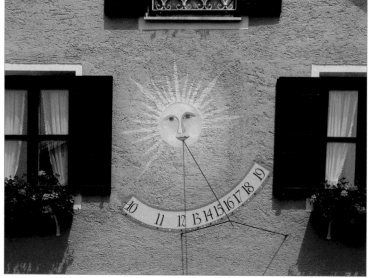

States means setting the clocks an hour forward on the second Sunday in March, then returning to standard time on the first Sunday in November. This "political time adjustment" has a similar effect on our bodies to "political time zones," except it also displaces our habitual rhythms by an hour, causing many people difficulties during the transition time. The organ clock, of course, remains aligned with the sun's movement and is unaltered by daylight saving time. Therefore, in places where daylight saving time is observed (all states but Arizona and Hawaii), when it is in effect we must also first subtract an hour from the time shown on the clock before calculating real time.

During daylight saving time, if it is used where you live, proceed as follows:

1. Correct for daylight saving time (subtract one hour from daylight saving time)
2. Calculate real time (as explained at the beginning of the chapter)

Now you know how to calculate real local time and can use the organ clock with a high degree of precision.

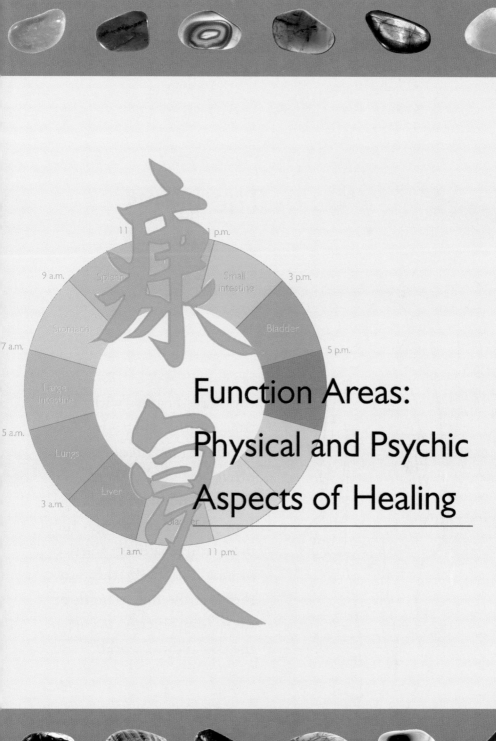

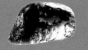   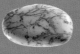 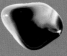

Function Areas:
Physical and Psychic
Aspects of Healing

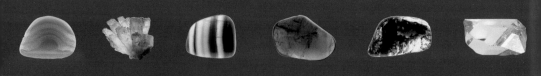

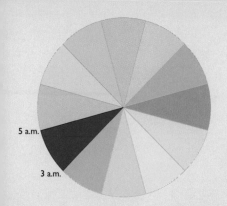

5 a.m.

3 a.m.

The Lungs

✦

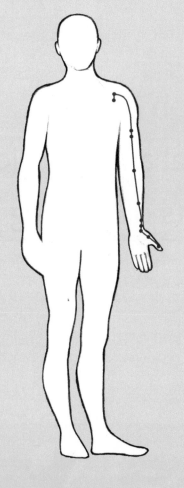

FROM THE CHINESE PERSPECTIVE, the day begins with the time of the lungs. In Zen Buddhist monasteries monks often rise at 4:00 a.m.—at the high point of the lungs' time—in order to begin the day with breathing practice or meditation. In this way, they use the full strength of their lung energy to meet the day and the world.

Lung meridian

32

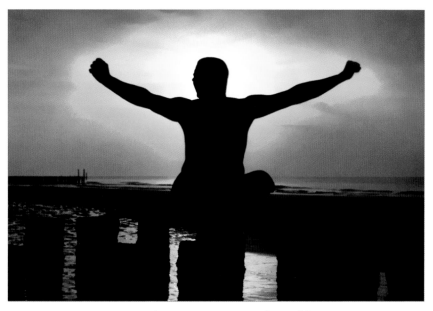

Breathing—connection to the world

BREATHING AND RECEIVING

The lungs take in the *chi*—the life energy that surrounds us and connects us with the world—and lead it into the body. This takes place through breathing, which is the most important function of the lungs.

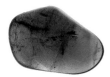

Amethyst releases feelings of closeness in the chest. Breathing thus becomes freer and deeper. Amethyst also promotes the exchange of gases in the lungs.

Apophyllite releases inner pressure and anxiety, helps with shortness of breath, and facilitates the intake of life energy. It's an effective healing stone for asthma.

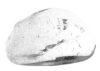

Aquamarine energizes breathing and intensifies the intake of life energy. Helpful for allergies affecting the air passages and restricting breathing.

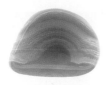

Blue chalcedony helps for respiratory illnesses and impurities in the air passages (smoking, pollution). Improves breathing function through self-cleansing of the airways.

Fluorite helps to resolve patterns of thought and behavior when they restrict personal freedom and block the natural life flow. Thus chronic tensions are released (and also chronic dry cough) and breathing becomes freer.

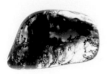

Moss agate helps with debilitating psychic pressure and bodily illness (infections, allergies) that lead to constriction of the air passages.

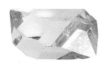

Rock crystal (quartz) opens the nose and upper air passages, makes breathing freer, and strengthens the flow of life energy.

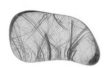

Rutilated quartz helps with anxiety and apathy, thus releasing tension in the chest. Imparts a feeling of breadth and greatness, deepening the breathing and increasing the volume of air inhaled. Helpful for bronchitis and lung blockages.

RHYTHMS OF THE BODY

Breathing, beginning with a baby's first cry and ending only with death, is—together with the heartbeat—the most dependable and most important rhythmical function of the body. The energy of the lungs is central to all the rhythms that determine life. This is true for everything from regular, strong breathing, to the pulse, to the rhythms of sleeping and waking. An irregular life rhythm (for example, a constantly changing work schedule) weakens the lungs.

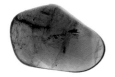

Amethyst calms the breathing, which also allows it to become deeper. Amethyst helps to achieve a regular flow in life, including time for composing oneself and for inner rest. Improves sleep and feeling of being awake and conscious during the day.

Apophyllite encourages openness to changing perceptions and needs when these have been suppressed by too much regulation. Supports confidence in the flow of nature.

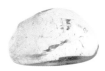

Aquamarine helps to regulate confusion and chaos, thus bringing rhythm back into life. Also helps with respiratory illness and allergies, which tend to stir up chaos in the body.

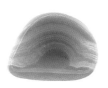

Blue chalcedony and **moss agate** facilitate harmony between internal rhythms and the rhythms of nature. Also helpful for sensitivity to weather, seasonal changes, jet lag, and temperature sensitivity.

Fluorite promotes regular life rhythms and restores order from disharmony brought about through irregular life changes. Makes all bodily rhythms more regular.

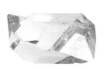

Rock crystal (quartz) encourages regularity in all bodily rhythms and brings them into resonance with natural rhythms, especially the alternation of day and night and the changing light levels of the seasons.

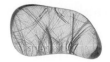

Rutilated quartz aids rhythmic bodily function and the rhythmic self-renewal of all cells, tissues, and organs. Also harmonizes spirit and soul with the rhythms of body and nature.

CONTACT AND CLOSENESS

The energy we receive through affection and devotion is every bit as important as the energy we receive from the air we breathe. Contact and closeness—both physical and psychic—influence and strengthen the lungs. So it is no wonder that the skin, our greatest organ of contact, corresponds to the lungs. All bodily hair is part of the skin function area, as are the sweat glands.

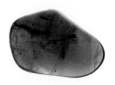

Amethyst helps alleviate the sadness that comes from the (danger of) loss of contact and closeness. Brings about inner peace, and helps with opening to the world once again. One of the best healing stones for the skin (itching, acne, eczema, and other skin diseases).

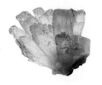

Apophyllite improves the ability to make contact by helping us to see ourselves as we are, without concealment, restraint, or a guilty conscience. Encourages the regeneration of skin and mucous membranes.

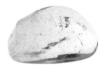

Aquamarine offers serenity in contact with others, and helps cure skin ailments resulting from allergies and autoimmune diseases.

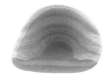
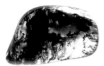

Blue chalcedony and **moss agate** facilitate openness and availability for contact, and promote cleansing of skin and mucous membranes.

Fluorite resolves behavior patterns that restrict our ability to make contact, and helps with tough, dry, or itchy skin.

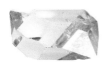

Rock crystal (quartz) makes us open and capable of contact; promotes skin functions and strengthens skin, hair, and nails.

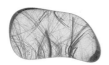

Rutilated quartz overcomes apathy and anxiety that originate from too little contact or affection. Encourages receptivity and courage. Also helps with sexual problems that result from fear of contact and estrangement.

COMMUNICATION AND EXCHANGE

Contact and touch are directly connected to openness and interest in other people. One of the most important functions of the lungs is their role in the ability to communicate: approaching others, speaking with them, and making ourselves understood—but also listening and understanding.

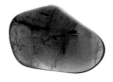

Amethyst promotes fair and just exchange on all levels. Helps to dissipate overly high expectations of others, thus protecting from disappointment. Strengthens lung function and helps heal lung ailments.

Apophyllite helps with open and honest communication as well as with conscious decisions as to what should and should not be imparted. Makes it easier to approach others and address them. Helpful for various air passage problems and diseases.

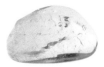

Aquamarine helps with the initiative to approach others, and to become acquainted and understood. Also helps, when necessary, for asserting verbally. Alleviates ailments of the neck, larynx, and vocal cords.

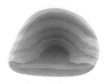

Blue chalcedony promotes joy in communication and contact; strengthens the ability to listen and understand, as well as the capability to express understandably. Helps with loss of voice, stuttering, and hoarseness.

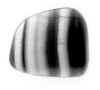

Fluorite encourages free expression, especially when others are trying to impair and restrict communication. Makes us quick-witted and easily understood. Also helps for coughs, throat pain, and respiratory illnesses.

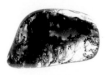

Moss agate promotes interest in surroundings. Helps with approaching others freely and overcoming obstacles. Relieves burdens on the soul, and throat problems such as coughs and "lumps in the throat."

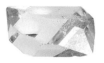

Rock crystal (quartz) facilitates clear expression and imparts a good sense for the right moment and words in communication.

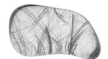

Rutilated quartz helps with various communication problems, alleviates fear and shyness about contact, and enables speaking freely and openly. Also helps with stage fright or beliefs about being too small, insignificant, or weak for self-expression.

DEFENSE

Sweating is one of the skin's important functions. From the Chinese point of view, the body's ability to sweat is connected with defense from illness. The lungs bear the major brunt of the body's defense: they are the first bulwark against disease, as well as against external bodily and psychic afflictions. As long as the lungs are strong, a person will not become ill.

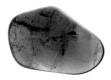

Amethyst, through inner peace, helps immunity against outer attacks. Regulates sweat secretion, whether too much or too little sweat.

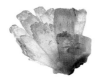

Apophyllite helps with psychic oversensitivity and with allergies, which are symptomatic of an oversensitive immune system.

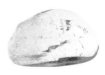

Aquamarine begins to diminish excessive sweating and overreactions of the immune system, such as autoimmune diseases and allergies, especially hay fever.

Blue chalcedony and **moss agate** cleanse the skin, thus easing sweating. Strengthens the immune system; especially helpful with respiratory infections.

Fluorite helps to protect against bodily and psychic afflictions and to remedy their aftereffects. Strengthens the immune system, especially in the skin and air passages.

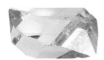

Rock crystal (quartz) strengthens the immune system, alleviates fever, and regulates sweating, whether too much or too little.

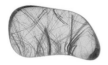

Rutilated quartz is helpful when lung function has been weakened through grief or anxiety, resulting in chronic illness (for example, chronic bronchitis).

NOSE AND SMELL

Another aspect of sweat is its smell. Someone's body odor is the most important factor in attraction or repulsion, and therefore is instrumental in determining whether contact will take place. The nose and sense of smell—and therefore the ability to evaluate "sweat information"— are closely connected to the function area of the lungs.

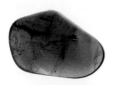

Amethyst improves the sense of smell but also helps with accepting smells of all kinds and tolerating them if necessary.

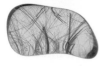

Apophyllite and **rutilated quartz** can restore lost sense of smell.

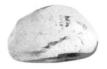

Aquamarine helps in being able to ignore smells and to remain uninfluenced by them.

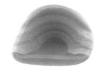

Blue chalcedony and **moss agate** improve the sense of smell by cleansing the mucous membranes of the nose.

Fluorite helps in tolerating strong smells and avoiding people who are "stinkers."

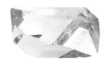

Rock crystal (quartz) improves the sense of smell and brings awareness of the impulses that arise from smell signals.

DISTURBANCES IN LUNG FUNCTION

Excessive lung function manifests psychically as a defense against any form of closeness. It is associated with issues of rigidity, control, and perfectionism. Physically, it can emerge in the form of oversensitive skin or allergies (overly strong defense).

When lung function is weakened, this is expressed externally in the form of skin, lung, and respiratory diseases (from slight colds to chronic asthma), and in general weakening of the immune system. The body's ability to take in energy is impaired, which can lead to a feeling of listlessness, weakness, or fatigue. Psychically, lung weakness can lead to an inability to make contact, or in the opposite case, to continuously come too close—an inability to respect and stay outside other people's boundaries.

Many of the stones that are suitable for lung support address both excessive and suppressed function, therefore recommendations for both are listed here.

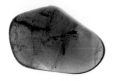

Amethyst supports respecting boundaries and over-coming sadness and lack of contact. It is the best healing stone for skin complaints (itching, acne, eczema, skin diseases).

Apophyllite helps with excessive lung function, as in allergies, asthma, fear of closeness, and psychic oversensitivity.

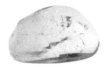

Aquamarine counteracts feelings of listlessness, weakness, or fatigue, and improves the ability to make contact. Also helps with loss of control and overreaction of the immune system, as in allergies and autoimmune diseases.

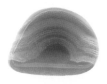

Blue chalcedony promotes contact, exchange, and communication. Improves the cleansing of skin and mucous membranes, and helps with respiratory ill-nesses and impurities in the air passages.

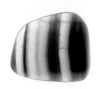

Fluorite improves the ability to make contact and release psychic defenses. Helps with rigidity and con-trol issues, and with persistent respiratory and skin ailments.

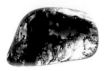

Moss agate facilitates communication, helps im-mune weakness and respiratory illness (infections, allergies). Promotes cleansing of skin and mucous membranes.

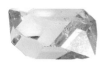

Rock crystal (quartz) brings energy in the case of being tired and weak, facilitates openness and abil-ity to make contact, and promotes skin functions.

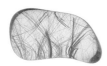

Rutilated quartz helps with weakness arising from grief and anxiety, the inability to make contact, and chronic respiratory illnesses (for example, chronic bronchitis).

STRENGTHENING THE LUNGS

Every kind of contact, physical touching, and regular rhythmic practice—such as breathing sessions or t'ai chi—will have a strengthening effect on the lungs. Cigarette smoke should be avoided.

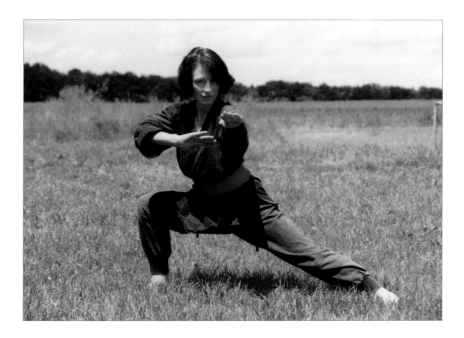

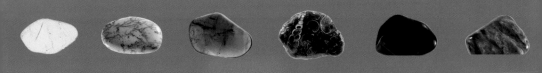

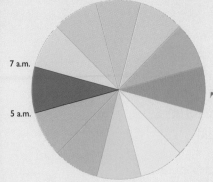

7 a.m.

5 a.m.

The Large Intestine

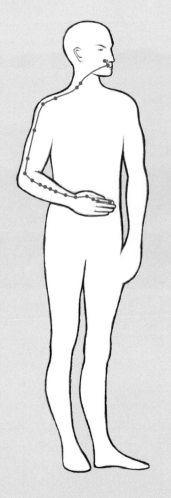

THE LUNGS' TIME on the organ clock is followed by the large intestine. Physically, intestinal cleansing takes place through the morning passing of stool. Additionally, the conscious morning ritual of washing—freeing oneself from sweat and nighttime secretions—is connected to the function area of the large intestine.

Large intestine meridian

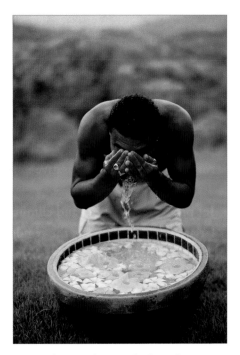

Washing—the ritual of purification

ELIMINATION AND CLEANSING

The main function of the large intestine is the active elimination of substances that are no longer useful. Besides the elimination of waste through the rectum, this also relates to all the body's cleansing functions (with the exception of elimination of liquid waste through the kidneys). Elimination through the skin in the form of perspiration also belongs to the function of the large intestine. The aspect of sweating, which helps purify the body, therefore belongs to the large intestine (while the aspect of contact and "reaching out to others" belongs to the lungs).

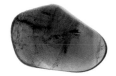

Amethyst improves elimination through the large intestine and skin; in both cases, it has a balancing function. Helpful for both diarrhea and constipation, as well as for excessive or insufficient sweat production.

Black tourmaline (schorl) is helpful for constipation and slow-moving bowels, releases tension and cramps, and speeds elimination through the large intestine.

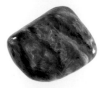

Charoite stimulates all elimination processes and promotes effective cleansing both in the living environment and, in the figurative sense, in all of life.

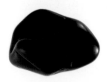

Jet promotes cleansing and elimination through the large intestine; supports the regulation of intestinal flora. Especially helpful with diarrhea.

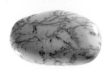

Opalite promotes cleansing of connective tissues, mucous membranes, and intestines. Promotes elimination functions and self-cleansing of the large intestine.

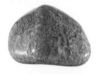

Pink moss agate stimulates digestion, elimination, and intestinal function; helpful for flatulence, diarrhea, and constipation. Improves gut flora.

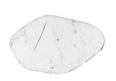

Spodumene (kunzite) is helpful when nervous complaints hinder the elimination functions of skin and intestines. Helpful for both too much and too little sweat, as well as for both constipation and diarrhea.

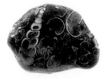

Turitella jasper improves elimination in the large intestine; frees the intestines from harmful contaminants (for example, heavy metals) and from trapped accumulations.

LETTING GO

The function of the large intestine encompasses not only bodily but also spiritual and psychic cleansing. The large intestine's function area disposes of both physical and psychic waste. Connected with this is the ability to let go of disappointment, hurt, and pain, which can burden and poison a person just as intensely as accumulated bodily waste.

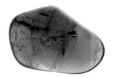

Amethyst helps with working through experiences and impressions, and letting go of them. Generally releases all kinds of attachments, thus bringing about a general inner cleansing. Amethyst has a psychically clarifying, lightening, and liberating effect. This also becomes obvious in the clarification of dreams, where it erases persistent images and creates new free space in the mind.

Black tourmaline (schorl) has a general relaxing, pain-relieving, and loosening effect. Enables letting go of negative thoughts, stress, and pressure.

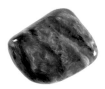

Charoite helps in dealing actively with psychic encumbrances and getting them resolved. Also relieves cramps and pain.

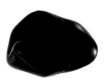

Jet helps in overcoming and releasing anxiety, sadness, and disappointment. Can also be helpful for inner emptiness and feeling unhappy for no apparent reason.

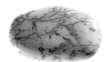

Opalite enables dealing with and accepting the moods and feelings of others. Especially helpful when excessive sadness becomes burdensome and inhibiting.

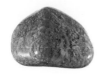

Pink moss agate enables letting go of uncomfortable memories and feelings of disgust, repulsion, vindictiveness, resentment, and combativeness, thus achieving openness and freedom.

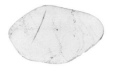

Spodumene (kunzite) promotes self-reflection, as well as letting go of hurt and pain. Also helps in finding the balance between self-criticism and self-acceptance.

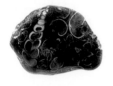

Turitella jasper is useful for letting go of burdens and negative experiences of all kinds. Also raises the power of resistance against environmental pressure.

SADNESS AND RELIEF

The ability to let go is especially important on the level of interactions between people: letting go of children as they grow up and move out, separation from friends or life partners, or even the death of a loved and trusted person. Letting go and turning loose, the great and small good-byes in life, are all within the domain of the large intestine. The ability to trust, release, and finally find relief or even redemption is one of the most important cleansing mechanisms in humans and is often our only option for finding inner peace after a loss.

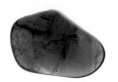

Amethyst helps in overcoming sadness and pining, including everyday disappointments: rejected attempts at contact, feelings of longing and alienation, unsatisfied yearning, partings, phases of separation. Amethyst encourages crying in order to find relief. It makes it possible to achieve inner peace, and supports the acceptance of unalterable circumstances.

Black tourmaline (schorl) brings neutrality and calmness, and generally eases letting go and releasing on all levels.

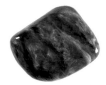

Charoite helps in getting through drastic changes in life. Eases parting and separation, turning the view forward. Especially effective with attachments to the past and with unresolved sadness from long-ago losses.

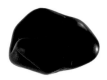

Jet is helpful with crises and lasting depression. Changes pessimism into confidence and trust; especially helpful when there is a lot to complain about but little initiative to change things.

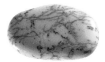

Opalite eases separations, and above all helps in letting go of whatever is not truly needed in life.

Pink moss agate enables resolution of unconscious mechanisms of stubbornness and persistence, and approaching life playfully.

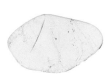

Spodumene (kunzite) teaches submission and humility and breaks down resistance, engendering a lighter mood and feeling of liberation.

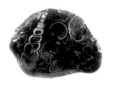

Turitella jasper helps us to withdraw from an excessive amount of responsibility, tasks, and engagements, and to consider our own wishes and needs without a guilty conscience.

PURITY AND OPENNESS TO NEW THINGS

After a parting has been entirely accomplished, a feeling of deep, inner purity remains. Separation and saying good-bye to old constructs (the

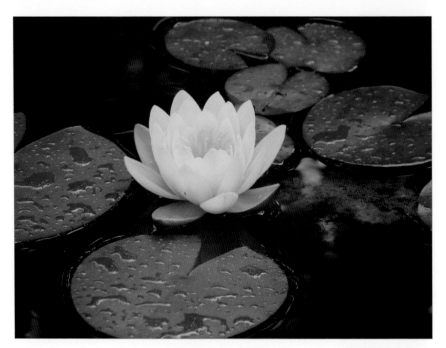

Undisturbed purity

large intestine) makes it possible to open up to new experiences, adventures, and meetings (the lungs).

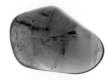

Amethyst offers purity through sadness, weeping, and letting go.

Black tourmaline (schorl) enables immediate, spontaneous letting go when uncomfortable experiences, pain, or burdens arise. Helps to preserve the feeling of inner purity, even in difficult situations.

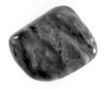

Charoite encourages opening to new ideas and experiences through active completion and cleansing of obsolete constructs.

Jet helps in expanding to include new things after long phases spent without any hope for improvement.

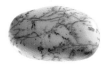

Opalite helps overcome fear of intimacy in the soul and psyche, and helps in reopening to surroundings and fellow humans.

Pink moss agate brings purity through strong elimination of both bodily and psychic baggage, which in most cases go hand in hand.

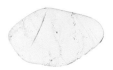

Spodumene (kunzite) brings joy to contact after long periods of withdrawal, and alleviates fear of possible hurt and disappointment.

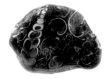

Turitella jasper, through distancing and inner reflection, helps to eliminate fear and guilty feelings. Thus leads to confidence and new openness.

DISTURBANCES IN LARGE INTESTINE FUNCTION

The elimination function of the large intestine can be either too strong or too weak. If it is too strong, this leads on the physical level to diarrhea; nourishment is expelled before it has been properly processed. On the psychic level, this often manifests as apathy—the feeling that everything is slipping away.

If the elimination function is too weak, the physical response is constipation. In the case of long-term weakness of the large intestine, waste accumulates within the body, overwhelming the organism with its own bilge. This leads to feelings of distension, bloating (there may be flatulence, but this is not always the case), and a general blocked or full feeling. When the large intestine malfunctions, the body endeavors to expel its toxic contents through the skin. This can result in extremely strong-smelling, pervasive sweat, or in skin diseases such as rashes, eczema, or acne. Extreme disturbances in the elimination process eventually will also affect the function area adjacent to the large intestine: the lungs. The consequences can be chronic colds, bronchitis, or asthma.

Psychically, a weak large intestine leads to cramplike stubbornness, because the affected person is unable to let go of what is no longer needed. This includes phenomena of compulsive preparation against all possible occurrences, as well as the inability to change the mind or step away from a certain viewpoint. Another effect of this weakness is that the process of grieving and letting go cannot be completed. Unresolved grief in the long term leads to depression, one of the most serious forms of large intestine weakness.

As with the lung function area, the stones recommended for healing the large intestine function have properties that address both excessive and suppressed function, therefore both are listed here.

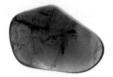

Amethyst regulates the eliminations of the large intestine, whether it is functioning too strongly or too weakly. It prevents the body from having to use the skin as an "emergency exit," thereby improving body odor and relieving skin ailments. By encouraging better psychic elimination, amethyst supports being open, awake, and conscious.

Black tourmaline (schorl) improves the elimination function, and helps with constipation and slow bowel function. Helps in letting go of psychic encumbrances such as negative thoughts, stress, and pressure; contributes to spiritual and physical flexibility.

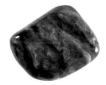

Charoite is useful for apathy and with the feeling that everything is beyond control, or that nothing can really be changed. Helps in understanding that losing and letting go do not "just happen," but take place through active interactions.

Jet helps with hopelessness and compulsive clinging to things long past. Makes changing perspective, and hence life change, possible again. Helpful for chronic large intestine blockage.

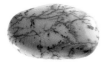

Opalite helps to track down toxic substances and eliminate them through the large intestine. Also cleanses connective tissue, skin, and mucous membranes.

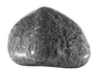

Pink moss agate supports releasing everything that is not absolutely necessary. Also resolves any compulsiveness and adherence to unconscious patterns. Consequently it is the most effective healing stone for slow bowel function, constipation, and flatulence, as well as for diarrhea. Also alleviates infections in the intestinal tract.

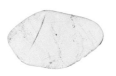

Spodumene (kunzite) is helpful for depression resulting from unresolved sadness, possibly bringing memories of the situation in question to the surface. Encourages flexibility in changing opinions and viewpoints, while still remaining true to self.

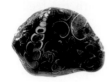

Turitella jasper loosens deposits resulting from too weak elimination, bringing about self-cleansing of the large intestine. Also helpful for compulsive clinging to negative experiences and perceptions, especially feelings of guilt.

STRENGTHENING THE LARGE INTESTINE

With an overactive large intestine, all spicy foods should be avoided. However, in the case of a weak large intestine, a good diet that includes hot spices is helpful (though not too much at first). Lots of exercise in fresh air will improve the condition of both large intestine and lungs. Here the emphasis should not be on effort but rather on endurance.

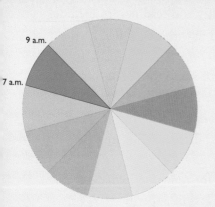

9 a.m.

7 a.m.

The Stomach

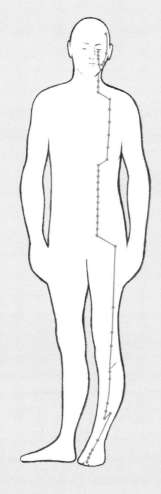

AFTER CLEANSING, IT IS TIME TO increase nourishment in order to gain energy for the day's work. That is why breakfast is the richest meal of the day in Buddhist monasteries.

Stomach meridian

55

RECEIVING AND ASSIMILATING

The stomach is for assimilating. This refers not only to the body's ability to digest nourishment but also to the ability and readiness to include something, engage in an effort, and deal with new things in life.

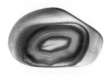 **Agate** fosters a feeling of safety in facing life and experiencing new things. Physically, it strengthens the stomach and digestion, and helps when worries (hard-to-digest thoughts) disturb the stomach.

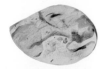 **Amber** creates appetite for new experiences and is also helpful for physical loss of appetite.

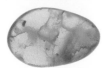 **Calcite** promotes the spiritual ability to receive and to be open to new experiences, and strengthens the stomach's digestive function.

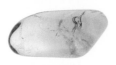 **Citrine** arouses the desire for change, new experiences, and self-realization. Stimulates active engagement in life and fulfillment of responsibilities. Correspondingly, also revives stomach function.

 **Dravite tourmaline** pacifies the stomach and strengthens its functions. Helps in opening to those around us and to new experiences.

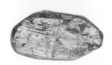 **Imperial topaz** helps in feeling secure and self-aware and in facing all new experiences. Brings great appetite and strengthens the stomach and digestion.

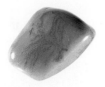 **Jasper** (brown and yellow) increases capacity for acceptance, as well as the stomach's productivity. Stimulates absorption of nourishment.

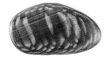

Petrified wood calms hectic activity, encourages pausing to "catch a breath," thus encouraging openness and assimilation. Eases pressure on the stomach and digestion.

TASTE AND PLEASURE

Biting, chewing, and swallowing—the entire process of eating—is necessary to be able to take in something. Therefore, the mouth, saliva, and sense of taste all belong to the function area of the stomach. Taste gives the first impression of the quality of the meal to be taken in and is often an indicator as to whether the nourishment is healthful and digestible. Analogously, the function area of the stomach is used for handling things in keeping with one's own tastes, allowing in only those things that "taste good" and that really do us good.

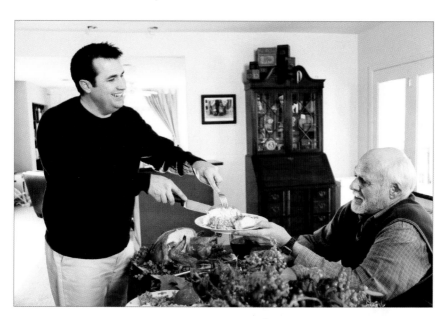

Enjoying a meal

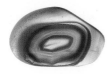

Agate regulates the composition of the saliva and improves the sense of taste. Stimulates enjoyment of food and good digestion.

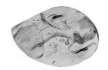

Amber creates the conditions for being able to bite and chew well, by strengthening children's teeth (teeth belong to the kidneys and bladder, but growth and development belong to the stomach and spleen).

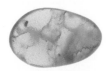

Calcite brings joy to eating and life, as well as a good sense of what is nourishing and agreeable.

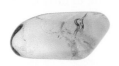

Citrine encourages thorough enjoyment of life and all it has to offer. This stone also helps relieve feelings of fullness—whether from overeating or for those who tend to feel full immediately after eating, regardless of the quantity consumed.

Dravite tourmaline helps to change harmful eating habits and correspondingly to develop "better taste" in food and in life.

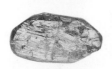

Imperial topaz encourages self-realization and creation of the life we desire. Helps in developing a good sense of one's own taste. Important healing stone for strong aversion to eating.

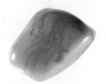

Jasper (brown and yellow) brings about pleasure in eating and the ability to appreciate simple fare. Gives a feeling of sufficiency and contentment with life.

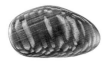

Petrified wood helps in accepting life and taking pleasure in earthly existence. Also stimulates enjoyment of eating.

NEEDING AND WANTING

The function area of the stomach not only supplies us with nourishment but also serves for the satisfaction of our psychic needs. If these cannot be fulfilled, the wish to possess something is awakened, or— more urgently—the feeling that one *must* have something. In extreme cases, this can lead to addiction or obsession.

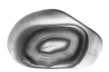

Agate supports the fulfillment of psychic needs, which leads to contentment and inner stability.

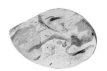

Amber encourages accepting things that are good without provoking an onset of guilty feelings. This condition leads to a feeling of having everything and needing nothing.

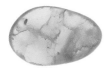

Calcite brings balance between having enough and wish fulfillment. Helps in obtaining the heart's desire.

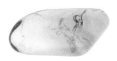

Citrine encourages ample satisfaction of needs and living out of desires.

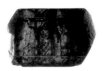

Dravite tourmaline is helpful for excessive hunger or an overly strong impulse to "have to have" things. Helps to satisfy real unfulfilled needs and to let go of false substitutes.

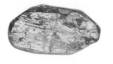

Imperial topaz clarifies recognition of what we already have (experiences, abilities, ideas, material possessions) and supports building on this basis to create more out of what is already present.

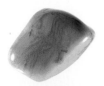

Jasper (brown and yellow) promotes the fulfillment of bodily and psychic needs, invigorating and strengthening.

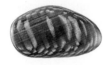

Petrified wood promotes simplicity and sufficiency, but without renouncing the pleasures of life. Helps in recognizing what is sensible and necessary without dragging along what is superfluous.

STABILITY AND REST

When all needs are fulfilled, rest and contentment follow. Having everything we need leads to calm and internal strength. We're not easily perturbed but work as a center of stability in our society.

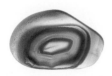

Agate promotes inner stability, calm, and a sense of community in relation to the immediate social environment (family, friends, groups). It brings balance to the energies and forces that flow in us. Encourages simple, pragmatic actions carried out with inner contentment and calm.

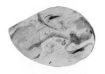

Amber encourages facing life in a calm and relaxed manner. Promotes a sunny attitude, coming across as gentle and compliant, yet being very self-aware.

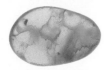

Calcite helps with self-confidence, stability, and perseverance; supports growth and maturity.

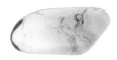

Citrine brings confidence and promotes a fundamental inner joy in living, based on a deep-seated sense of security.

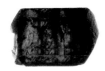

Dravite tourmaline inspires serenity, calm, and contentment. Promotes a sense of community, readiness to help, and social engagement.

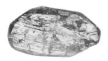

Imperial topaz produces a feeling of inner wealth leading to a serene, secure demeanor and the ability to encourage and support others along the way.

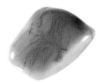

Jasper (brown and yellow) is helpful for mastering life by doing what needs to be done (no more and no less).

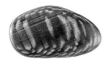

Petrified wood promotes grounding, rootedness, and a feeling of being at home anywhere on the planet. Guides us to be in the right place at the right time, and to be firmly rooted in reality.

NOURISHMENT AND FUEL

For a community to survive, it is important to take care of children and weaker members. The stomach meridian runs through the nipples and physically influences milk production. In general it is responsible for the ability and willingness to take care of others and provide what they need in life. People who share what they have create a pleasurable effect in others. Sympathy is an expression of the function area of the stomach.

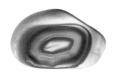

Agate helps in making others comfortable. Useful during pregnancy and as a protective stone for mother and child; stimulates milk production in nursing mothers.

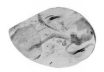 **Amber** strengthens our nurturing side and encourages devotion to others, caregiving, and support. Confers magnetism and sympathy.

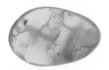 **Calcite** inspires giving energy to the community, especially encouraging children in their development. Makes milk richer in nutrients.

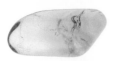 **Citrine** stimulates extroversion and an interest in other people. Can promote lively social engagement when there is an inclination for it.

 **Dravite tourmaline** promotes readiness to help and sense of community by sharpening perceptions of the needs of the social environment.

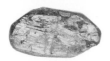 **Imperial topaz** helps in nurturing and taking care of others on the impetus of inner feelings; also stimulates productivity. Fosters open-mindedness and generosity.

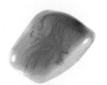 **Jasper** (brown and yellow) promotes social engagement and energetic commitment to the community. Fosters sharing with the community.

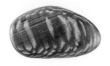 **Petrified wood** encourages being rooted in the community, sheltering and nurturing others like a great tree. Enables simply being present for others when they need someone.

DISTURBANCES IN THE STOMACH

An excessively strong stomach function area makes one want, or even need, to have *everything*. This results in the loss of the ability to distinguish between what does good and what does harm. People with this affliction stuff themselves indiscriminately without being able to digest properly or evaluate what is ingested. Such a person has constant strong needs that are difficult to truly satisfy, since what is taken in is not what actually is needed. In its advanced stages, this problem manifests as increasingly strong cravings, ultimately leading to addiction.

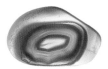

Agate offers contentment and a feeling of sufficiency, promoting recognition of what really is and is not needed in life.

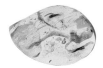

Amber is helpful when too much food has been indiscriminately "gulped down," both physically and psychically. Helpful for melancholy, nausea, and stomach complaints.

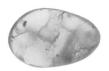

Calcite helps to distinguish what will do good from what will cause harm, and to evaluate all the useful components of nourishment. Stimulates growth and promotes psychic and spiritual development through a good evaluation of life's requirements.

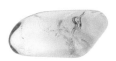

Citrine helps in processing a surplus of images (for example, negativity in the media), and to get rid of pressures that have accumulated. Correspondingly, helps with excessive or substandard food intake leading to a full feeling or an upset stomach.

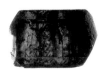

Dravite tourmaline is helpful for growth problems due to malnutrition. Has a balancing effect when needs are either too strong or severely suppressed.

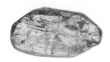

Imperial topaz increases perception of what has already taken place, drawing contentment from the vast wealth of experience. This makes clearer what is still needed, causing superfluous needs to disappear in the continued effort to create a rewarding life. Also guides in proper evaluation of food and gaining a few pounds if there is a need.

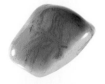

Jasper (brown and yellow) improves the evaluation of nourishment that is absorbed. Fosters contentment with simple living conditions, causing frivolous desires to vanish.

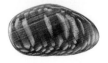

Petrified wood diminishes the desire to have everything that seems enticing. Helpful in losing excess weight that is caused by lack of grounding or excessive appetite.

When the function area of the stomach is too weak, the intake of nourishment is not guaranteed. This leads to deficiencies (both in food and in psychic necessities) and to a feeling of being unable to provide for oneself. Someone with these weaknesses is not able to receive what is needed for life. Energy is low, exhaustion comes quickly, and there is a tendency for lethargy and apathy. It's not possible to absorb all the things that come up, meaning there is a lot "left on the plate."

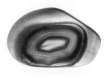

Agate assists in taking in and processing whatever is really necessary for life. Promotes the well-balanced intake and digestion of psychic impressions.

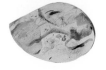

Amber is useful for stomach upset and nausea, especially when there is too much "on the plate."

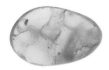

Calcite helps to balance out nutritional deficiencies and strengthen the stomach when digestion is weak. Also has a psychically strengthening effect, and helps to turn ideas into reality.

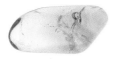

Citrine stimulates digestion when the stomach lacks strength to process food. Psychically assists taking in external impressions better and more quickly.

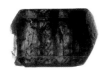

Dravite tourmaline supports taking good care of self and others. Provides sufficient energy without strain. Strengthens the stomach and helps with stomach upsets.

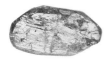

Imperial topaz imparts the feeling of being able to take good care of self and others. Brings energy; helpful for lethargy and apathy.

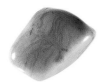

Jasper (brown and yellow) strengthens those who are easily exhausted; promotes stamina and endurance. Increases stomach function.

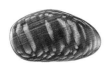

Petrified wood brings stability, grounded energy, and interest in life. Encourages taking good care of self and being present for others. Helpful for deficiencies.

STRENGTHENING THE STOMACH

The basis for strengthening the stomach is healthy, adequate nutrition. In general, this should consist of about 75 percent whole grains and vegetables, supplemented by other fresh foods and a little meat or fish. All addictive substances—especially caffeine and flavor enhancers—should be avoided as much as possible.

Centering body exercises, such as t'ai chi and qi gong, also have a strengthening and balancing effect on the stomach.

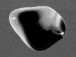

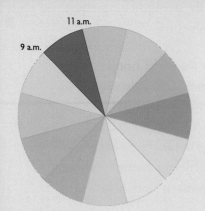

The Spleen

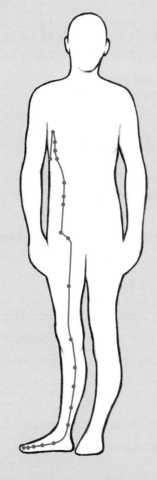

ONCE THE INTAKE OF nourishment has been completed, the day's work begins. The spleen's role in the body is that of a worker, and this time of day corresponds to the carrying out of everyday labor.

Spleen meridian

MANAGEMENT AND DISTRIBUTION OF ENERGY

The spleen draws in the life energy (chi) contained in the nourishment drawn in by the stomach and distributes it to all the other function areas. The spleen regulates this distribution so that each function area, at any given time, is always receiving exactly what it needs. The spleen's task is the management of resources.

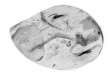

Amber ensures that supplies will be distributed and not simply stockpiled. Promotes generosity with the resources available and helps to manage them for constant abundance.

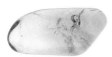

Citrine promotes good overall distribution of energy (this is easily perceived when it is placed on the abdomen). Has a generally stimulating effect, raising energy level by improving the absorption of energy from food.

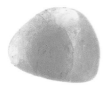

Golden beryl ensures a goal-oriented distribution of resources, so that life energy is applied sensibly and not squandered, but also is not held back.

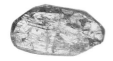

Imperial topaz improves the ability to build resources and share them generously. Gives a feeling of having limitless energy, by allowing access to unused forces and abilities.

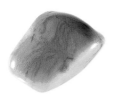

Jasper (brown and yellow) helps to draw energy from food and to store up energy reserves; these constantly well-stocked reserves provide endurance and inner stability.

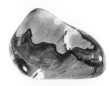

Mookaite brings flexibility so that energy distribution is optimally tailored to the situation. This keeps the entire system in equilibrium.

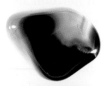

Sardonyx stimulates cell metabolism and body fluids; promotes absorption of nourishment and decontamination of tissues.

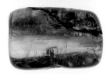

Yellow tourmaline promotes good energy distribution and releases blockages that impede distribution.

HARMONY AND COORDINATION

The spleen enables the function areas to work together. It regulates task division and cooperation among different parts of the body. By channeling the chi through the body, it ensures that the organs remain in their own places and do not shift or prolapse. The spleen is responsible for the harmony of body and soul, and therefore for the harmonic functioning of the whole person.

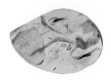

Amber promotes harmony, well-being, and good cooperation among all areas of life. Fosters feeling truly good in one's own body. Also optimizes metabolism and provides for, and strengthens, connective tissues.

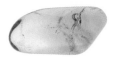

Citrine has a slight stimulating effect on all function areas, restoring movement to dormant spheres of life and leading to an exhilarated, dynamic, active feeling of wellness.

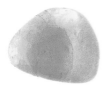

Golden beryl strengthens all the coordination functions of the nervous system: the nerves of the senses (for remaining in control), the motor centers of the brain, the motor nerves for movement coordination, and the vegetative nervous system as a regulator for the interplay of the internal organs. It's also helpful for nausea and other coordination problems arising from stress.

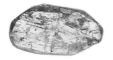

Imperial topaz promotes good internal and external coordination. Stimulates nerve function and makes the organism more reactive and adaptable to new situations. Assists harmonious entry into new situations.

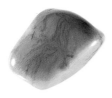

Jasper (brown and yellow) tightens and strengthens the whole body, promoting the supportive function of connective tissues and thus working against shifting and prolapsing of internal organs. Promotes good cooperation among the internal organs and gives a feeling of well-being throughout the body.

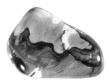

Mookaite helps external activities and internal processing of their results to remain in balanced equilibrium.

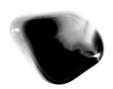

Sardonyx promotes harmonious energy distribution throughout the body, adjusting for surpluses and deficits. Also helpful with energy imbalances resulting from stress.

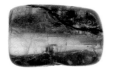

Yellow tourmaline coordinates the entire interplay of the internal organs, and improves coordination between body, soul, intellect, and spirit.

CHANNELING THE BLOOD

The spleen function area distributes and directs the blood, keeping it on its course. It controls the connective tissues, nourishing them, keeping them strong, and channeling bodily fluids. The spleen also supplies the sex organs with blood and moisture, thus making sexuality and fertility possible.

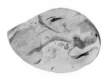

Amber keeps connective tissues elastic and stimulates the body to cleanse them and provide them with nourishment. Supports the functions of the sex organs and promotes fertility.

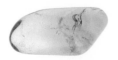

Citrine has a stimulating effect on the sex organs and awakens interest in lively sexuality.

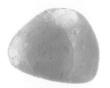

Golden beryl improves the interplay of all organs, and also regulates blood flow so that each organ is supplied optimally.

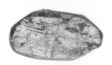

Imperial topaz enhances fertility and the ability to enjoy sexuality. Generally promotes pleasure.

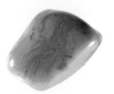

Jasper (brown and yellow) improves supply to connective tissues and distributes energy to the limbs in order for them to be well supplied. Helpful for feelings of heaviness in the limbs and associated joint problems.

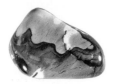

Mookaite promotes and harmonizes circulation, so that blood goes to where it is needed. Improves blood quality and wound healing.

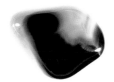

Sardonyx guides the blood by strengthening blood vessels and assuring that the blood stays in its channels. Promotes good circulation and blood supply to connective tissues, as well as higher blood quality.

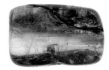

Yellow tourmaline supports finding fulfillment in sexuality by strengthening the sex organs and the harmony of body, soul, and spirit.

LEARNING FROM MISTAKES

The function area of the stomach serves for the intake of nourishment and psychic impressions. The spleen function area is responsible for processing these things. Its task is to digest food and work through experiences. The ability to learn from mistakes and integrate them as experience into one's life is the most important outcome of this process.

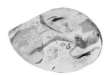

Amber assists in avoiding becoming unsettled by mistakes, making new attempts, and believing in self. Consequently eases the path to success.

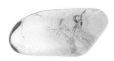

Citrine improves the spiritual digestion of the impressions received, so that mistakes will not be repeated. Likewise improves physical digestion.

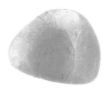

Golden beryl facilitates working through experiences, drawing conclusions from them, correcting mistakes, and actively changing consequences. Also helpful for various digestive problems.

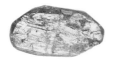

Imperial topaz integrates experiences easily and quickly, and reveals errors as opportunities for improvement. Also strengthens and reinforces digestion.

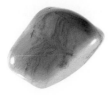

Jasper (brown and yellow) helps for remaining undaunted after failure, and trying again until the difficulty is overcome. Brings collectedness and inner peace for carrying out plans sensibly. Correspondingly, helps (symbolically) to "bite the bullet."

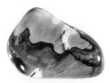

Mookaite reveals more and more possibilities, but assists in making the right choice without any trouble. Regulates spleen function and improves digestion.

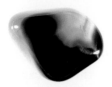

Sardonyx promotes a virtuous character in terms of social rules; thus leads to endeavoring to avoid mistakes and behave "correctly." One of the most important healing stones for spleen ailments.

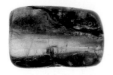

Yellow tourmaline stimulates interest in correcting mistakes. Promotes the general wish to get things in order, as well as a good sense of what is not in order.

COMPREHENSION

A balanced, strong spleen supports comprehension. The foundation of harmony is the ability to recognize what is needed and to evaluate the consequences of every decision. This in turn leads to fulfillment and happiness.

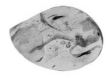

Amber improves the perception of needs that must be fulfilled *immediately*. Brings almost endless success: assists in being in the right place at the right time, so that everything "just works."

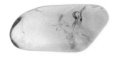

Citrine improves understanding through direct observation and the pragmatic use of things already known. Leads swiftly to fulfillment and happiness.

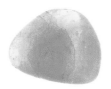

Golden beryl brings continuous, comprehensive understanding. Increases effectiveness: things are thought through to the end, and all necessary details for achieving a goal are taken into consideration.

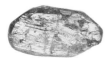

Imperial topaz offers a broader comprehension in that it helps for seeing the whole and recognizing the right place for all things. Shows what must be done so that all things can unfold in their natural order. Helps for arranging these things.

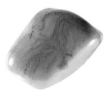

Jasper (brown and yellow) isolates what is truly needed. Confers the ability to evaluate consequences simply but unerringly.

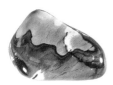

Mookaite promotes a wish for change and new experiences. Also brings inner peace and a desire for adventure; deepens the realization that meditation is possible in every task.

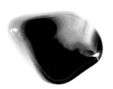

Sardonyx improves perception of *real* requirements, that which is truly needed, not just what is desired. Illuminates the consequences of actions and promotes working toward harmonious development.

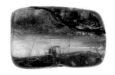

Yellow tourmaline enables interpreting the meaning of specific experiences—recognizing what these have brought and for what good purpose.

DISTURBANCES IN THE SPLEEN

An excess in spleen function leads to the quick exhaustion of bodily resources and malnourishment, as well as the inability to gather reserves. It results in a strong tendency to have allergies, since the immune system is not balanced. In the psychic domain, it is expressed as chronic discontent, imbalance, and inner restlessness. This often leads people into harmful thought circles, spiraling thought patterns from which they cannot escape. Excessive spleen function—or sometimes a weak spleen—can also lead to a tendency toward grouchiness, or to criticize self and others constantly.

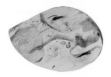

Amber promotes a sunny, positive, worry-free attitude in life. Helps for gathering energy and building up reserves. Instills contentment and balance, and calms thought circles. Also helpful against allergies.

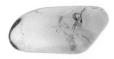

Citrine banishes melancholy and downheartedness, and puts life in a positive light.

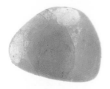

Golden beryl promotes sensible distribution of energies, thus offering amazing stamina that can "move mountains" and the ability to work for long periods without rest. Also alleviates allergies.

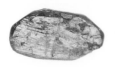

Imperial topaz is restorative for exhaustion caused by stress; it strengthens the nerves. Stimulates the appetite and helps people who "can't do anything." Positive effects for anorexia have also been observed.

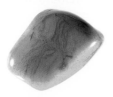

Jasper (brown and yellow) helps conquer exhaustion resulting from lack of resources, and promotes equilibrium and endurance. Strengthens tolerance, attending to personal concerns, and not perceiving others as irritating.

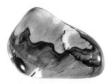

Mookaite stabilizes health and forestalls a sickly condition. Remedies conditions of weakness, strengthening the immune system. Helpful for allergies resulting from long-lasting disorder or confusion.

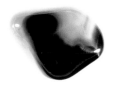

Sardonyx is very effective against allergies. It helps to cure illnesses completely, leaving no basis for allergies and complications to emerge. Encourages a complete cycle to end. Cycles pertain to the change phase of the earth.

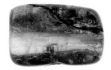

Yellow tourmaline brings happiness and content-ment; dispels ponderousness, grouchiness, and critical attitudes by bringing full acceptance. Instills benevolence and understanding.

A weak spleen results in a deficiency in the processing of food and expe-riences alike. In the case of food, the body is not adequately nourished and becomes sickly and weak. The blood does not stay in its channels, which easily leads to bruises or to heavy and irregular menstrual flow. Tissues are weak, flabby, and possibly waterlogged. The function areas do not work together harmoniously, so there are energy blockages and congestion. The extremities (hands and feet) are cold, because blood and chi do not make it to the tips of the fingers and toes.

Psychically, this weakness manifests as timidity, melancholy, insecu-rity, and indecision, or else indifference. Learning from experiences is very slow, meaning that the affected person has a strong tendency to repeat past mistakes.

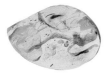

Amber enlivens the whole body, pervading every cell with spiritual energy. Leads to affirmation of the body and of life.

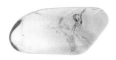

Citrine improves the processing of nourishment (digestion) and of experiences; brightens mood and brings courage to face life.

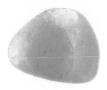

Golden beryl conveys self-assurance, confidence, and decisiveness; helpful against timidity, melancholy, and indecision. Facilitates learning quickly from experiences.

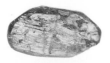

Imperial topaz has a mood brightening effect, promotes self-awareness, and helps prevent nervousness and stage fright.

Jasper (brown and yellow) strengthens a weak spleen; tightens and tones connective tissues.

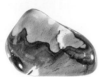

Mookaite remedies lack of experience by conferring a sense of adventurousness and confidence to try new things. Encourages embracing life in all its many forms.

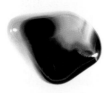

Sardonyx makes menstrual flow more regular, neither too strong nor too weak. Reinforces blood vessels (protection against stroke) and improves circulation in tissues. Awakens interest in life and interaction with other people. Counteracts feeling dull; opens all the senses, and stimulates enjoyment with all the senses!

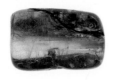

Yellow tourmaline brings happiness and contentment; strengthens confidence in innate abilities.

STRENGTHENING THE SPLEEN

Besides the indications for nourishment given for the stomach, the best way to strengthen the function area of the spleen is to create a secure space in which to simply be one's true self. It is also important for children and people in long-term partnerships to have space that is theirs alone.

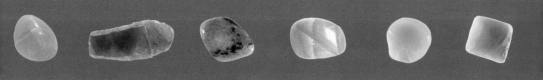

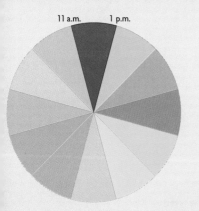

11 a.m.   1 p.m.

The Heart

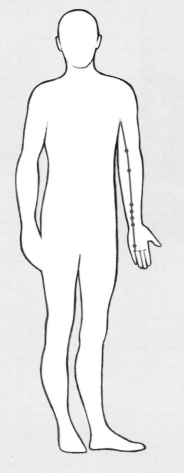

THE TIME OF THE HEART is also a time of rest. Many people feel the need to lie down at this time (especially if they are early risers) and take a midday rest. The reason for this is that the heart's main time of activity is a span in which feelings should be put into words, and this is best done while undisturbed.

Heart meridian

77

RULER OF EMOTIONS

In Chinese medicine, the heart is connected with emotions, and especially with love. Its strongest function is to feel empathy with others and to want to stand by them. The heart governs the emotions, which in turn are crucial in determining how each individual will experience and perceive the world.

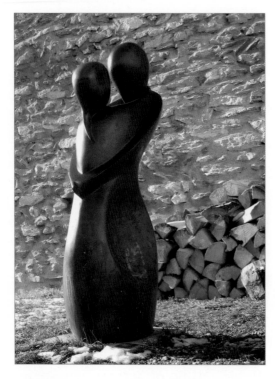

Empathy and support

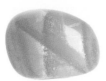

Moonstone intensifies feelings, improves perception of them, and helps in following intuition, which is the "voice of feelings."

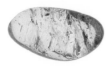

Morganite supports perceiving and accepting emotions as essential parts of life, also making it possible to express feelings. Awakens a love of life and of all living things.

Pink chalcedony promotes well-being and heartiness, imparting worry-free, calm, deep confidence. It opens the heart to the world, strengthening the ability to listen and to help others overcome their problems and worries.

Pink opal promotes impartiality and generosity toward others and an easygoing attitude. It shakes off shyness, shame, and inhibitions.

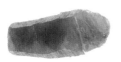

Pink sapphire encourages all-embracing love of the world and all beings, without demands or possessiveness, full of acceptance and readiness to help.

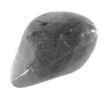

Pink tourmaline encourages tenderness and affection, and eases the way for other beings and for connection with them. Confers outgoing charm and warmheartedness, placing the wish to receive in harmony with the ability to give.

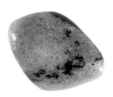

Rhodonite heals hurt feelings and promotes forgiveness, self-acceptance, and self-love. Strengthens empathy for all beings.

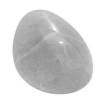

Rose quartz strengthens empathy and perceptiveness. Encourages self-love, strength of heart, romance, and ability to love.

SEAT OF THE SPIRIT

The task of the heart function area is to govern the body via the brain and the five senses. The heart is the body's central authority and the seat of the *shen* power, which is purely spiritual energy and can be viewed as a person's true nature. The brain is an organ subject to the heart, simply serving to convey its intentions to the body. The Chinese word for heart (*xin*) means simply "center" and describes what truly makes up a person's innermost nature.

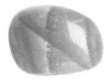

Moonstone allows one's true nature to rule, even when the intellect wavers among different options and directions.

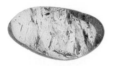

Morganite helps in laying out the tasks set in life and in wholehearted dedication to achieving them. Brings awareness of excessive psychic needs.

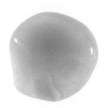

Pink chalcedony brings liveliness, understanding, and readiness to help. Teaches how to see the world with wondering eyes and promotes natural curiosity and readiness to meet with the world and all beings openly, and to learn from them constantly.

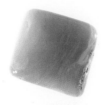

Pink opal helps in holding to higher ideals and acting altruistically. Provides an inner connection of spirit, soul, and body, so that both psychic wishes and bodily needs can be satisfied.

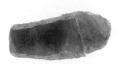

Pink sapphire strengthens the spirit so that it can put both the inner and outer worlds in order. Helps in doing all things with love.

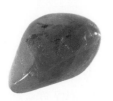

Pink tourmaline makes connections among body, soul, and spirit, so that all aspects of life are joined and are oriented toward spiritual intention. Consequently helps in living as an individual being from the inner life and in active dedication to life tasks.

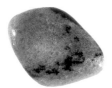

Rhodonite strengthens the shen, or ability to be as one is. Consequently helps the heart to preserve its function as a central power, even in extreme situations. Maintains clarity and consciousness in situations of shock, harassment, or high pressure. Also good physical protection for the heart.

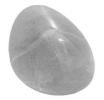

Rose quartz brings greater fulfillment from efforts, and support for remaining on the right path in life. Assists in not living "outside of oneself" and in fulfilling life and heart wishes.

BLOOD AND VITALITY

The heart's function is to rule the blood and blood vessels and to maintain a strong, stable pulse. The strength of the heart is synonymous with a person's vitality. It determines all of our active expressions, such as heartiness and enthusiasm, as well as the intensity with which we take part in the world and in the game of life.

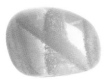

Moonstone strengthens participation in life and the world, and thus intensifies perceptions, sensations, and experiences.

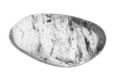

Morganite promotes interest in the game of life. Strengthens and reinforces the heartbeat, but quiets an overly fast pulse. Aids regeneration, strengthening the heart and increasing vitality, preventing possible exhaustion.

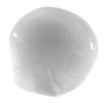

Pink chalcedony strengthens the heart so that it can work powerfully but without straining. Brings liveliness, but also calms excessive activity and tension.

Pink opal makes the heart strong, flexible, able to respond to strain quickly, and able to return to quiet equally quickly. Infuses enthusiasm and vitality, and raises the intensity of life.

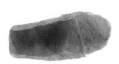

Pink sapphire intensifies experience and preserves identity. Improves personal control over life and promotes generous clarity in dealings with others. Provides solid, sustainable vitality and a strong, stable heartbeat.

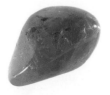

Pink tourmaline inspires dynamism and flexibility, and promotes healthy, adaptable vitality. This is manifested in a strong, free blood flow, an adaptable heartbeat, and a healthy, resilient heart.

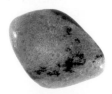

Rhodonite strengthens the heart so it can endure heavy strain. Brings vitality and a life force that is all the more enduring for not being ostentatious. Stabilizes circulation, making it an excellent stone for healing wounds.

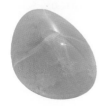

Rose quartz sets the heart in the right rhythm and balances its function so that it remains enduringly strong and vital. Equalizes activity and rest into a constantly sustainable balance.

LANGUAGE AND LIFE

"The heart opens to the tongue," traditional Chinese medicine tells us. This means that the ability to speak is synonymous with the ability to speak to others, to inspire them, and to move them to work with us. The heart is the seat of the spirit, a person's true self. And this spirit, in turn, makes itself understood through speech and expression. He who can speak openly shows himself to all others, not making his heart into a den of thieves.

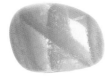 **Moonstone** helps with insightful expression and an ability to find the "right words" (or "right silence") in either joyful or sad situations.

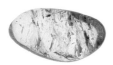 **Morganite** supports being engaged and dynamic, and also helps with letting go of excessive ambition and fanaticism. Promotes a warmhearted authority to which others gladly turn. Helps in expressing things clearly and directly without causing hurt.

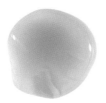 **Pink chalcedony** improves the capacity for confident, heartfelt communication. Helps solve conflicts openly and honorably; also makes us somewhat loquacious.

 **Pink opal** resolves downheartedness and worry, makes us hearty and hospitable, and loosens the tongue. The maxim "He whose heart is full, his mouth runneth over" can be applied to pink opal.

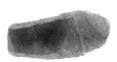 **Pink sapphire** promotes love of truth and helps with clear and direct expression that is also careful and gentle, so that nobody gets hurt. Strengthens the power of persuasion, which is the ability to reach others with words.

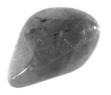 **Pink tourmaline** makes us outgoing, charming, lovable, and affectionate. Helps us to "touch" others, motivate them, and speak heart-to-heart.

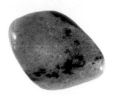

Rhodonite helps in expressing things that are deeply affecting due to sadness, pain, or hurt, allowing an unburdening of the soul. Rather than making us talkative, it helps with formulating what is really relevant. This leads to a healing of the heart and aids in reconciliation between people who have hurt one another.

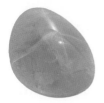

Rose quartz stimulates approaching others openheartedly and warmly. Makes us gentle, but in keeping with the motto "The soft and weak overcomes the hard and strong."*

GOOD SLEEP AND SPIRITUAL HEALTH

Another function of the shen, the heart's spiritual aspect, is a relaxing, healthy night's sleep. Someone whose heart function area is strong and balanced will sleep quietly and deeply. This leads to spiritual peace, inner strength, and strong perceptions.

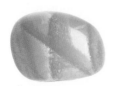

Moonstone improves sleep by bringing the inner rhythm of body and soul into harmony with the outer rhythms of nature. If there is a large discrepancy between inner and outer rhythms, this can lead to "primary aggravations" in the form of sleep disturbances. Moonstone helps in perceiving not only the outer manifestations of beings and things but also their inner expression.

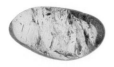

Morganite eases stress and performance pressure, encouraging time for leisure and tranquillity. Tensions vanish and sleep improves. Morganite brings inner calm, strength, and crystal-clear perception.

---

*Lao-tzu, *Tao Te Ching,* chapter 36.

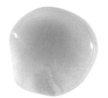

Pink chalcedony dispels worry and brings inner peace, great confidence, and consequently, deep sleep. Improves attentiveness and helps with perceiving finer nuances in both sight and sound.

Pink opal brings comfort, and thus good sleep. Also turns perceptions inward during the day, which may manifest as dreamy contemplativeness; in this process, many new ideas and concepts can emerge from wishes and memories.

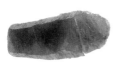

Pink sapphire encourages comfortable, sound sleep, even in unsettled or difficult times. Promotes clarity, inner peace, and strength; sharpens the senses; makes the mood mild and friendly.

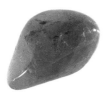

Pink tourmaline calms for balanced sleep during the night and a relaxed, attentive wakefulness during the day, without any stress.

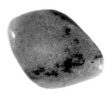

Rhodonite helps heal psychic wounds and scars, and supports forgiveness of hurt and injustice. Frees from psychic pain, fermenting anger, and persistent irritation. Helps us to "sleep the sleep of the just."

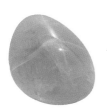

Rose quartz soothes the mind, thus producing good sleep, if our deeds and efforts are in harmony with our true spiritual intent. If we have deviated from this intent, it makes us restless until we recognize it and get back on track.

DISTURBANCES IN THE HEART

Excessive heart function makes us oversensitive and pitying. The latter does not refer to the ability to put ourselves in others' shoes and compassionately help them; this ability is known as empathy. Pity, on the other hand, is a form of hypersensitivity. A pitying person makes another's pain her own, suffering from the misfortunes of others. This extreme hypersensitivity weakens the heart and makes the affected person unable to find inner peace. Blood pressure rises, and heat and restlessness fill the body.

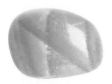

Moonstone promotes empathy, perceptiveness, and the ability to distinguish between one's own true opinions and invasive opinions. Prevents descent into pity; helpful for hypersensitivity. Has a cooling effect, also lowering blood pressure and calming in times of severe inner restlessness.

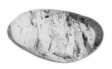

Morganite encourages changing pity into constructive empathy, and helping others when needed and possible. Relieves inner restlessness.

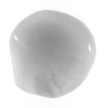

Pink chalcedony enables facing the misfortunes of others with understanding and readiness to help— without engendering clinginess. Helps with excessive sadness and a troubled heart (cardiac neurosis).

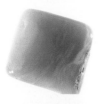

Pink opal helps in working through sadness so that it will lead to active empathy rather than pity. Calms inner unrest and allows heat to flow out.

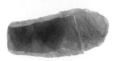

Pink sapphire stimulates empathy without any trace of pity. Fortifies consistency and "tough love" (therefore helpful for parenting). Relieves inner heat and restlessness, and lowers blood pressure.

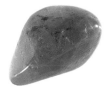

Pink tourmaline protects against people inviting pity or foisting unwelcome feelings on others. Watermelon tourmaline, a pink tourmaline with a green outer layer, is best for this. Pink tourmaline has a balancing effect on body heat and blood pressure.

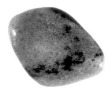

Rhodonite promotes self-love, and therefore is supportive in rising out of pity—a form of deficient self-love—to proper self-love wherein we do not take on others' suffering. Rhodonite strengthens the heart in all its functions: heartbeat, rhythm, and regeneration.

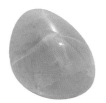

Rose quartz promotes empathy, perceptiveness, and readiness to help. Helpful for accelerated heartbeat and inner unrest, as well as high blood pressure when it is caused by a disturbance in the heart.

If the function area of the heart is too weak, this manifests in the form of impassivity and hardheartedness. Both are symptoms of a lack of feeling toward other people, which is synonymous with an inner retreat from the world and from society. Someone who loses contact with his heart will, in time, become solitary and lonely. Physically, a weak heart function area may lead to insufficient generation and control of blood. The consequences are low blood pressure and anemia.

Both forms of heart disturbance may influence the clarity of the mind, leading to confusion, hallucinations, and finally even to insanity.

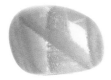

Moonstone improves the ability to empathize and our dedication to the world and dealings with others.

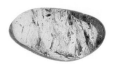

Morganite helps with impassivity and hardheartedness; helps to overcome self-importance and retreat from life's responsibilities. Promotes a clear mind and self-control in cases of confusion or mental illness.

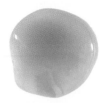

Pink chalcedony encourages turning toward others with warmth and generosity. Gently raises low blood pressure and supports the forming of blood.

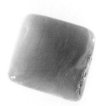

Pink opal promotes generosity toward others and involvement in the world and society. Strengthens the heart; helpful for many heart ailments, including cardiac neurosis. Raises low blood pressure and improves blood production.

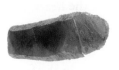

Pink sapphire brings spiritual clarity and promotes a desire for knowledge and wisdom, which seeks fulfillment not in isolation but in all of life. Therefore also promotes social engagement as a manifestation of active empathy.

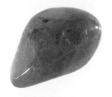

Pink tourmaline warms the heart with patience and love. Strengthens openness and devotion and connection to other beings. Promotes blood cleansing and blood formation.

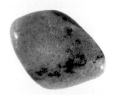

Rhodonite encourages empathy, understanding, and forgiveness, and helps in mediating quarrels. Heals old pain and enables preservation of mental clarity, even in extreme situations. Stabilizes the heart and circulation, promotes blood formation, and eliminates shock.

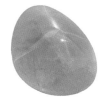 **Rose quartz** sharpens perception by bringing good intuition and the ability for deep empathy. Brings awareness of forgotten needs, thus bringing body, soul, and spirit into connection. Helpful for a weak heart; also balances out disturbances in heart rhythm.

STRENGTHENING THE HEART

The heart is best strengthened by rest. Overloading, performance demands, stress, pressure, and a fast-paced lifestyle all damage heart function to a great degree. A regular midday rest period during "heart time" is one of the best ways to restore equilibrium.

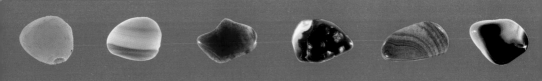

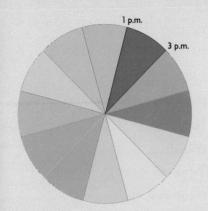

1 p.m.

3 p.m.

The Small Intestine

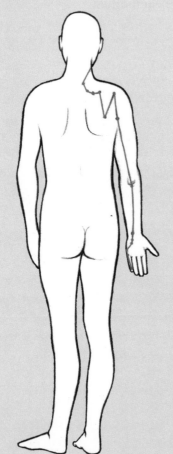

AFTER THE TIME OF THE HEART COMES the high point of activity in the inner world; many people take an afternoon nap, or at least an afternoon break, during this time. These two hours are especially good for allowing thoughts and inner images to surface and enter into dialogue with wishes and goals.

Small intestine meridian

FILTERING AND SORTING

The main task of the small intestine function area is filtering. It sorts the nourishment that is taken in and determines which components are useful and which must be expelled. Physically, it separates food-stuffs from waste. On the psychic-spiritual level, it fosters the ability to distinguish things from one another—to recognize what's what. Consequently the small intestine helps us to work through experiences and to acknowledge our own goals and wishes.

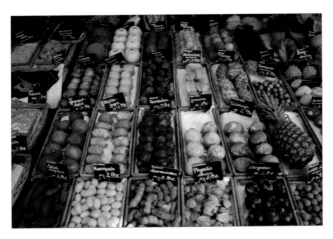

Good sorting

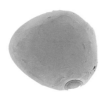
Carnelian generally improves the absorption of vitamins, nutrients, and minerals in the small intestine, and thus imparts vitality and liveliness. Psychically, it offers the courage to open to new experiences and challenges.

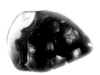
Fire agate is helpful for disturbances in small intestine function following illness, infection, and ingesting bad food. Also useful in working through bad psychic experiences, learning from them, and developing a positive worldview from them.

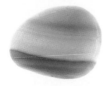

Manganocalcite gently stimulates digestion and improves nutrient intake. Improves the ability to discriminate; improves reflection (the ability to distinguish memories from each other).

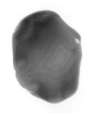

Pink agate stimulates the intake of nourishment into the intestines and helps with nausea, infection, and irritable bowel syndrome (functional disturbance in the intestine without organic illness, often stress related). Instills new confidence in bad situations.

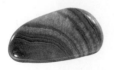

Red agate strengthens the small intestine and helps with food selection that confers energy and vitality. Also fortifies psychic endurance and energy for realizing goals and wishes.

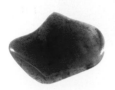

Red chalcedony reduces nourishment intake to the essentials, especially when the organism is inclined to take in too many unnecessary things. Also reduces spiritual perception and intent to the essentials, meaning goals and wishes are strengthened and an excess of impressions can be more easily processed.

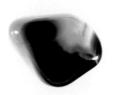

Sardonyx stimulates small intestine function and improves both nutrient intake and elimination. Promotes stable healthiness through a good selection of nourishment. Affords a better understanding of the meaning of things that happen from day to day.

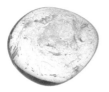

Topaz stimulates the small intestine to take in all that is needed from food; therefore, it is helpful for many kinds of deficiencies. Helps self-acceptance and the strength to claim and protect the space necessary to realize goals and wishes. Especially helpful for recognizing what truly belongs to us.

PERCEPTION

The ability to perceive something is fundamentally connected with the ability to differentiate. Thus, the intensity of perception is often coupled with the small intestine function area, even when—depending on the sense in question—other function areas also play a substantial role. The ability to pick out sounds and thus to understand what is being said is part of the function of the small intestine, even if the sharpness of hearing depends on the condition of the kidney and bladder function area.

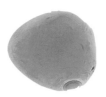

Carnelian makes us attentive and realistic. Helps avoid clouding perceptions with opinions and memories, so we are able to see what simply is.

Fire agate helps in reorienting negative perceptions and focusing on positive things. Encourages awareness of subtler nuances and reading between the lines.

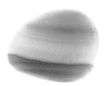

Manganocalcite promotes cooperation, loyalty, and acceptance; allowing perceptions in, rather than blocking them out due to fear or worry.

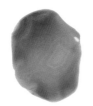

Pink agate promotes attentiveness, thus improving perception. Encourages thoughtful evaluation of impressions and new information, which leads to better understanding.

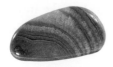

Red agate focuses attention on personal concerns, blocking out those of others. Assists us in reaching a goal of finding or researching something.

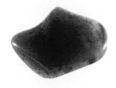

Red chalcedony in areas of interest offers intense attentiveness that defies distraction. This is the "watchman" of the healing stones, helping us to react swiftly to perceptions.

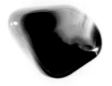

Sardonyx strengthens all the sense organs, improves receptiveness, and intensifies perception. Also helps with better processing and understanding of sensory perceptions.

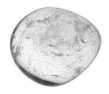

Topaz improves the ability to differentiate and perceive; especially helpful for a better understanding of things perceived by the senses. This makes it possible to gain wisdom from the turnings of fate.

ABILITY TO PERCEIVE THINGS

A person's ability to perceive things has a lot to do with how "good" feelings are distinguished from "bad" feelings. The small intestine enables us to see inside others, to tell how things are going for them, but not to lose ourselves or strain too much in doing so. In this manner, it enables us to protect our own boundaries without having to withdraw inward or become apathetic.

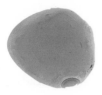

Carnelian brings openness to the feelings of others without the danger of being influenced by them. Carnelian strengthens a sense of community, as well as personal viewpoint.

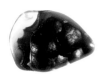

Fire agate assists in coming to terms with feelings, and above all in changing negative feelings. Also improves perception of others' feelings, and helps in distinguishing what is personal from what is foreign.

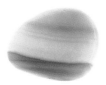

Manganocalcite improves the ability to perceive, and makes it easier to sense when someone else's perceptive ability is causing difficulties. This promotes friendliness and warmth between people.

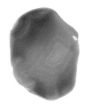

Pink agate promotes sympathy, at the same time helping to soften angry feelings. Helps keep us entirely in tune with others, yet still able to remain conscious of self.

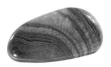

Red agate safeguards personal boundaries, and helps in deciding where to direct perceptive abilities and when to retract them. Protects sensitive people from being flooded by outside perceptions.

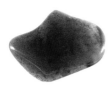

Red chalcedony helps for going along with others without forgetting our personal viewpoint. Enables protection of personal boundaries and respect for those of others.

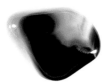

Sardonyx fosters friendliness and a readiness to help, while also enabling communication of feelings. Therefore, it promotes the ability to share positive feelings with others and lighten their moods.

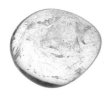

Topaz helps in protecting personal space and not getting drawn in by others' perceptions and moods. Also helps identify feelings.

DISTURBANCES IN THE SMALL INTESTINE

Excessive small intestine function leads to an inclination to hypersensitivity; on the spiritual-psychic level, this manifests as overloading. The ability to tell things apart is overwhelmed, so that it becomes impossible to distinguish one's own feelings from someone else's, or in extreme cases, to tolerate any feelings at all. Everything is too deeply affecting, and even when one is alone, it can all be too much.

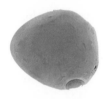

Carnelian improves digestion and helps with enjoyment of foods to which the small intestine usually reacts strongly. Brings stability, resilience, and self-support. Promotes a life-affirming view and an inner readiness to take on things that will be beneficial.

Fire agate is helpful for function disturbances and infections in the small intestine. Brings joyfulness and contentedness, lightens the mood, and helps us to avoid being influenced by other people's moods.

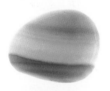

Manganocalcite calms the small intestine when it is irritated and sensitive. Helps in dealing with strain and brings joy to the emotional life, thus enabling open connection with others.

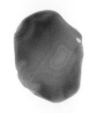

Pink agate is helpful for disturbances in the small intestine resulting from stress, hypersensitivity, and strain (irritable bowel syndrome). Calms emotional turmoil and helps us to find inner peace, confidence, and warm security.

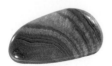

Red agate is helpful for hypersensitivity in the small intestine, especially when slight nausea regularly occurs a short time after eating. Fosters inner peace and establishes boundaries against other people's feelings.

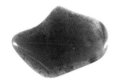

Red chalcedony halts excessive nutrient intake and diminishes feelings of hunger. Helps in overcoming difficulties and pressures, collecting thoughts, and establishing boundaries when things are overwhelming.

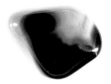

Sardonyx is helpful for infections and diseases of the small intestine, and for the effects of other illnesses (infections, allergies, immune weakness). Psychically, it promotes self-control and brings inner stability, self-reliance, and confidence.

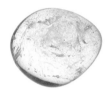

Topaz makes the small intestine resistant and stable, and soothes oversensitivity. Enables clear separation between what belongs to us and what does not. Helps us to endure emotions, accept them, and find fulfillment in them.

When the small intestine function area is too weak, it can no longer take in everything needed for living, growing, and thriving. It is no longer able to distinguish right nourishment from wrong, which leads to deficiencies and/or poisoning. Perceptions become less sharp, or in extreme cases become distorted, and it becomes very difficult to process events and experiences and integrate them into one's life. Suppressed small intestine function leads to lack of perception and consequently to numbing and lack of interest in the affairs of one's fellow humans.

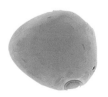

Carnelian improves nutrient intake and helps with deficiencies. Lends a sense of reality in confusing times, helps with processing experiences, and engenders openness and interest in other people and the environment.

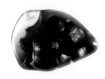

Fire agate stimulates regeneration in the small intestine after weakening illness and assists through unhappy events, helping to integrate them into life. Preserves perceptiveness and awakens interest and zest for life.

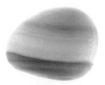

Manganocalcite enhances digestion and nutrient intake, as well as perceptiveness and interest in interactions with others.

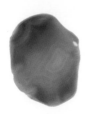

Pink agate improves nutrient intake and helps remedy deficiencies caused by using up reserves too quickly, for example in the case of infection or other illness. Helps in working through difficult experiences and maintaining interest in other people.

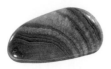

Red agate strengthens the small intestine in cases of extreme weakness and improves nutrient intake. Helps keep perceptions clear, and promotes a lively interest in other people and surroundings.

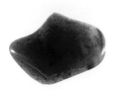

Red chalcedony influences taking in only what is needed from food, especially avoiding poisoning from malnutrition. Helps maintain a clear view, even in moments of weakness, and staying on track despite being overwhelmed by too many impressions.

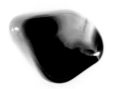

Sardonyx strengthens the small intestine, regulates deficiencies, and helps eliminate poisons. Clarifies and sharpens perception, and helps in processing experiences. Offers lively sensations and strong interest in other people and surroundings.

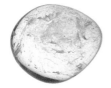 **Topaz** enables the small intestine to distinguish clearly what is needed from what is not. Strengthens food intake; especially helpful for deficiencies. Improves perceptiveness and the ability to gain farther-reaching knowledge from all kinds of experiences.

STRENGTHENING THE SMALL INTESTINE

Like the heart, the small intestine benefits from rest at the proper time of day. This rest does not have to be especially long; a mere five or ten minutes for closing one's eyes and allowing inner images to surface will work wonders. To simplify and strengthen the bodily intake of nourishment, it is advisable to set aside a short rest period (ten to fifteen minutes) after each meal, in order to digest and absorb food more thoroughly, rather than jumping back into work right away. This will benefit not only the small intestine but also the stomach.

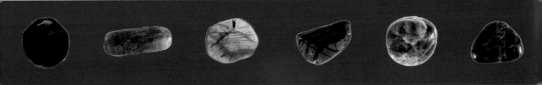

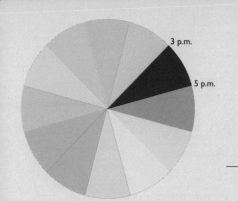

3 p.m.

5 p.m.

The Bladder

THE TIME OF THE BLADDER is another period of activity and strength for many people (when this is not the case, there is a disturbance). It is the best time of the afternoon for working effectively and getting things done.

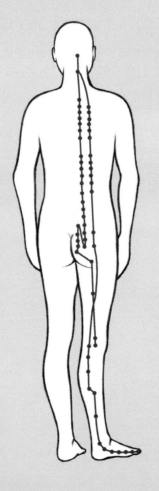

Bladder meridian

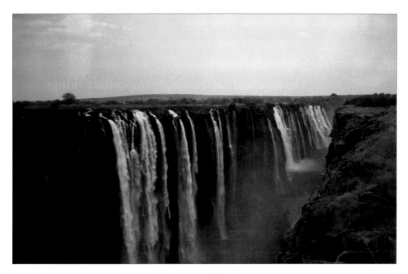

Power and energy

ENERGY AND CONDUCTIVE POWER

The kidneys—the partner function area to the bladder—are where a person's energy reserves are stored. The ability to put these reserves to use lies within the function area of the bladder. This is the area we draw upon when we accomplish something, not allowing ourselves to be discouraged or distracted by difficulties that arise. Assertiveness, and the ability to turn intention into action, are signs of a strong and healthy bladder function area.

 Blue apatite mobilizes energy reserves and brings new force, especially in times of exhaustion or after a burnout phase. Motivates and helps with being assertive.

 Blue tourmaline strengthens trust, ethics, and the courage to stand by deeply felt truths. Supports taking responsibility and doing what must be done.

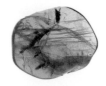

Cordierite (iolite) gives strong endurance and stamina even in the most adverse conditions. In extreme situations, it gives the spiritual force of will to accomplish seemingly impossible things.

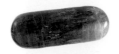

Kyanite strengthens the power of assertiveness, even in very difficult situations; supports an escape from fatalistic beliefs and victim roles.

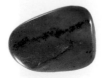

Lapis lazuli helps us to remain true to self and to go our own way honorably and sincerely. Supports advocating truth and fairness.

Pyrope garnet builds up the energy reserves of the kidneys, and increases self-determination and assertiveness. Strengthens force of will and vigor.

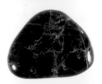

Sodalite strengthens idealism, the search for truth, and the will. It encourages being true to self in both concept and conduct.

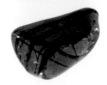

Sugilite supports being uncompromising in achieving a goal. Strengthens identity and will.

ABILITY TO ACT AND CONTROL

The ability to reach goals is synonymous with the ability to act according to our wishes and control our own lives. The ability to exercise control is one of the bladder's most important qualities. This can either be bodily control (the ability to stand upright corresponds to the bladder) or control over the conditions of life. Another important quality of the bladder is the ability to lead others and hence—taking things a step further—the ability to control them.

Blue apatite lends liveliness, motivation, and drive to put variety into life. Helpful against apathy and listlessness; prods slumbering ideas into action.

 Blue tourmaline promotes conscious dialogue with inner abilities, strengths, and weaknesses; therefore improves conscious control over life.

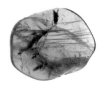 **Cordierite** (iolite) enhances psychic and physical performance and strengthens the spine, so that outside pressure will not cause collapse.

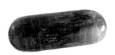 **Kyanite** releases outer pressures that feed on the will and life energy. Strengthens control over individual actions.

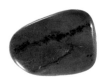 **Lapis lazuli** supports the mastering of conflicts and open expression of opinions. Lapis lazuli helps each of us to be ruler of our individual (spiritual) domain, and thus recognized as an authority.

 Pyrope garnet preserves the capacity to act, even in crises and difficult times. Improves control over living conditions.

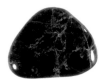 **Sodalite** imparts a clear feeling of identity; helps us make space to live a life chosen freely and consciously.

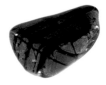 **Sugilite** keeps us competent even when external or internal demands threaten to consume us. Helpful for fear, paranoia, and psychic ailments; improves bodily control.

ADAPTABILITY AND SUCCESS IN LIFE

Effective advancement is possible not only through forcible imposition of personal will, but even more through adaptation to external conditions. The ability to remove hindrances, when this is possible and necessary, belongs to the bladder as well as the ability to adapt to conditions that cannot be changed. Having a combination of these two qualities makes it easy to achieve whatever is undertaken.

Blue apatite guides us to use our life energy more economically. Makes us goal oriented and successful through a proper distribution of force and spontaneous release of energy when necessary.

Blue tourmaline helps for being as "pliant and inexorable as water," always finding new ways and possible solutions when seemingly insurmountable obstacles emerge.

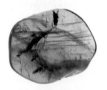

Cordierite (iolite) endows the ability to endure even the most unpleasant circumstances. Helps with avoiding senseless struggles and waiting patiently for the right moment.

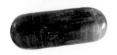

Kyanite brings calmness and resolute strength in situations where everything is going haywire. Balances logical, rational thought and spontaneous, instinctive action.

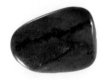

Lapis lazuli helps in accepting criticism, and contemplating and insightfully correcting a course of action when there is a justified reason for doing so. Consequently helps increase wisdom.

Pyrope garnet, in situations in which there is no hope or perspective, supports doing all that is necessary and going forward step-by-step until the crisis is overcome.

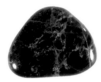 **Sodalite** confers awareness of thought and behavior patterns when they prevent us from acting or lead repeatedly to failure. Makes us successful and able to learn.

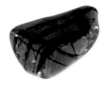 **Sugilite** helps for dealing with uncomfortable things without shying away, and finding conflict solutions that work toward unification and do not put anyone at a disadvantage.

DRIVE AND SURVIVAL

The bladder function area also takes over automatic control of the body when consciousness fails. Most subconscious regulating mechanisms belong to the bladder—reproductive urges, deeply rooted instincts,

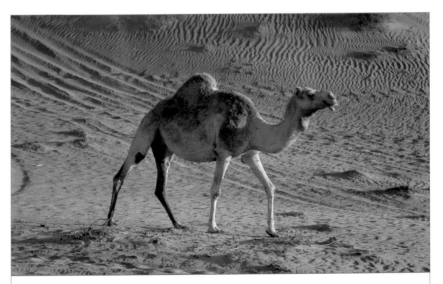

Survival artist of the desert

survival skills, and the hormone system that activates and regulates many of these survival mechanisms. Survival skill in itself is one of the bladder's most important functions; associated with this is the ability to endure pain and torment without giving up.

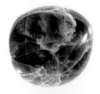

Blue apatite increases self-control and capacity to act despite exhaustion and depletion. Gets us back on our feet with an appetite to take in new energy.

Blue tourmaline intensifies unconscious reactions and improves the perception of involuntary impulses and drives. Improves water retention and regulates hormones. Alleviates pain; especially helpful for burns.

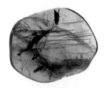

Cordierite (iolite) makes all bodily mechanisms function optimally and guarantees the necessary capacity to act. Strengthens to endure hardships and troubles, and alleviates pain and cramps.

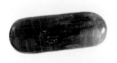

Kyanite, in emergencies, activates instinctive action in order to assure survival, but also preserves consciousness and self-control. Helps endurance of pain, agony, and extreme psychic low points.

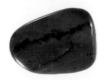

Lapis lazuli places individual survival before reproduction, and if necessary, suppresses the sex drive so that this energy can be directed into other domains of life. Also slows hormone cycles necessary for fertility (the menstrual cycle) while strengthening other hormone cycles related to individual productivity (the thyroid gland).

Pyrope garnet stimulates the will to survive and brings energy for fighting adversity. Stimulates the sex drive, eliminates inhibitions, promotes repro-ductive power, and helps with impotence.

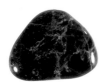

Sodalite promotes the optimization of unconscious regulation mechanisms by integrating conscious learning experiences. Regulates water retention and improves the functionality of the hormone system.

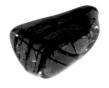

Sugilite confers an unswerving will to survive and overcome fears, and allows psychic intent to domi-nate unconscious reactions. Strengthens to endure suffering; has a strong pain-relieving effect, and amplifies the sex drive and hormone system.

DISTURBANCES IN THE BLADDER

Excessive bladder function often leads to an explosive personality, and in extreme cases to loss of control: instinct and drive become all-powerful, and the intellect can barely retain authority. Physically this manifests as intense restlessness and also a strong likelihood of a reced-ing hairline and baldness (although the reverse, that everyone who is bald suffers from excessive bladder function, is not necessarily true).

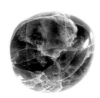

Blue apatite reduces irritability and aggression; helps with inner restlessness (and also hyperactiv-ity) and with bladder problems such as urine reten-tion or irritable bladder.

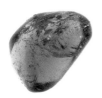

Blue tourmaline releases pent-up feelings, brings relaxation and inner peace. Makes us calm, tolerant, and clear in our understanding. Regulates water reten-tion and helps with almost all bladder problems.

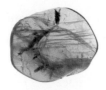

Cordierite (iolite) relaxes and calms an explosive temperament. Helpful for nervous bladder disturbances.

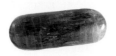

Kyanite helps for keeping under control and not becoming overwhelmed by surging emotions. Imparts flexibility and improves finger dexterity.

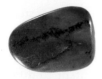

Lapis lazuli cools rage and helps to control anger (but without suppressing the cause, which is usually communicated immediately and bluntly). Helps in more conscious control of drives.

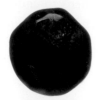

Pyrope garnet brings a calm feeling of security and strength. It is helpful for bladder complaints such as inflammation and infections.

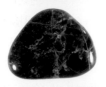

Sodalite keeps a cool head without suppressing feelings and inner impulses. Also helps control these through conscious observation. Regulates water retention and bladder function; helpful for urine retention and irritable bladder.

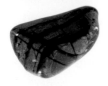

Sugilite releases psychic tension; helps to master fears and achieve inner balance. Strengthens self-control and even helps with manic episodes.

Suppressed bladder function leads to torpidity; if the bladder is too weak, the person loses the capacity to act. A typical expression of this is a victim complex—the feeling of being at the mercy of external conditions and having no control over life. Physically, severe bladder weakness can lead to incontinence.

Bladder weakness can also lead to opposite extremes and manifest in compulsive desire for control and ambition for power. Everything must be controlled and brought under the person's rule. It is important to understand that, as with all conditions in traditional Chinese medicine, exhaustion of the bladder could be hidden by extreme activity. This form of excessive bladder function arises when one cannot tolerate one's own weakness. The weakness is concealed by an energetic manner but is not remedied.

Blue apatite gives a boost out of bodily and psychic low points caused by the depletion of life energy (burnout syndrome), which lead to complete loss of control in life.

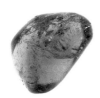

Blue tourmaline gets us back on our feet (in thoughts, emotions, and bodily functions) and loosens rigidity (symbolically, dried-up water) and desire for control (symbolically, stagnant water). Imparts confidence, security, and ease. Helpful for almost all bladder complaints.

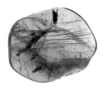

Cordierite (iolite) helps prevent ever losing control and the ability to act, even under rigorous circumstances. Also helpful for incontinence.

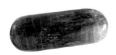

Kyanite helps restore lost control over life and the ability to act, ends feeling like a victim, and supports striving for self-determination. It generally improves body control and often helps with incontinence.

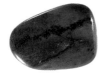

Lapis lazuli clarifies self-awareness and the ability to take life in hand. Also eliminates imperiousness and excessive desire for control.

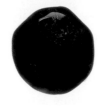

Pyrope garnet helps with both fearful rigidity that impairs the capacity to act and with excessive desire for control arising from fear of rejection and failure. In either case, it engenders confidence and security. Also helpful for physical bladder weakness and incontinence.

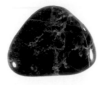

Sodalite frees blocked feelings and dissolves guilt. Encourages more freedom of expression and strengthens the ability to act. Generally alleviates compulsive behavior and the desire for control. Helpful for bladder weakness and incontinence.

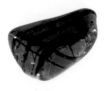

Sugilite dilutes debilitating rigidity arising from fear and unhealthy desire for control and power. Strengthens trust in self and loosens psychic cramping. Alleviates pain and helps bladder complaints and incontinence.

STRENGTHENING THE BLADDER

Enough sleep and plenty of water are best for strengthening the bladder. It is important to drink only pure, noncarbonated water in sufficient quantity (at least two liters every day). Rest periods should be times of real relaxation, not just a nap in front of the television.

The bladder is also improved by exercises that strengthen one's force of will; the best physical exercises for this are demanding but not too difficult and can be increased without becoming boring. Mountain hiking at various levels of difficulty is especially good for the bladder; so is swimming in a lake or ocean (but only very briefly in a chlorinated swimming pool).

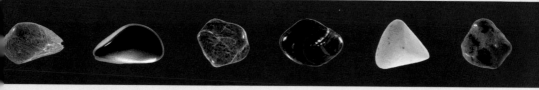

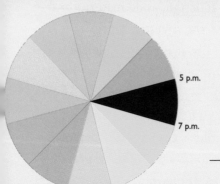

5 p.m.

7 p.m.

The Kidneys

◆

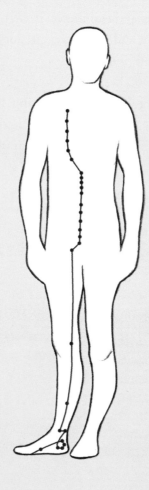

EVENING IS APPROACHING and it's time to end the day's work gradually. With the time of the kidneys, we begin to turn our attention inward to take care of personal needs and recover from the day's exertion.

Kidney meridian

111

INHERITED TRAITS AND CONSTITUTION

The kidney function area contains the beginning and end of life. The ability to reproduce belongs to the kidney function, as do maturity and old age. The kidneys are the seat of the *jing,* the ancestral energy that is passed on from parents to children. Physically, it is responsible for the human constitution: how strong we are, how much endurance we have, and how great is our resistance to disease.

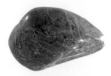 **Epidote** helps to rebuild a constitution depleted by overstrain, exhaustion, or illness; especially strengthens resistance to disease.

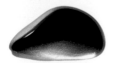 **Hematite** gives stamina and endurance, strengthens and reinforces the body, and helps to assure survival on all levels (bodily and psychic).

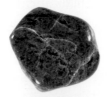 **Nephrite** brings inner balance, protecting from burnout and supplying reliable energy. Strengthens both physical and psychic constitution, even under pressure, stress, and strain.

 Obsidian mobilizes the spirit and helps in working through shock and traumatic experiences, which might otherwise lead to a breakdown of energy.

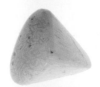 **Scolecite** gently and steadily strengthens the constitution; stabilizes productivity at a steady, high level.

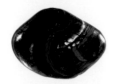 **Tiger iron** helps us use our potential to the fullest, mobilizing energies and abilities that may sometimes surprise us.

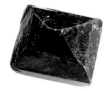

Zircon offers an indefatigable constitution, able to survive the most terrible situations—undefeatable!

Zoisite (with ruby crystals) regenerates after complete exhaustion or severe illness. Has a noticeable strengthening and reinforcing effect.

LIFE ENERGY

In addition to the ancestral jing energy, energy reserves we accumulate in life are also stored in the kidneys. The stronger the kidney function area is, the more life energy a person has to use. People who positively radiate energy, are never tired, and rarely need sleep have a strong and healthy kidney function area.

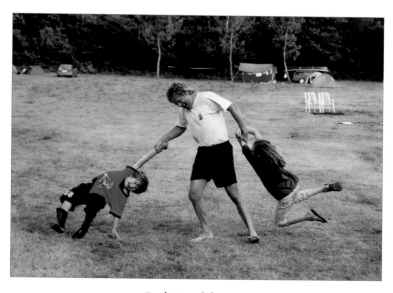

Radiating life energy

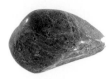

Epidote is helpful for lack of energy, yields strength and power, and assures that sufficient energy will constantly be available. Improves productiveness through optimal distribution of energy.

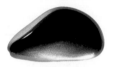

Hematite bestows energy, vitality, and liveliness; helpful for chronic fatigue and deep exhaustion. Gives a pronounced feeling of strength, and makes us dynamic and active.

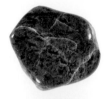

Nephrite makes us fit, lively, and productive, with a feeling of "solid energy" that is not aggressive but is available for use whenever needed.

Obsidian releases energy blockages and frees the flow of life energy. Has a strong, enlivening effect, banishing fatigue and weakness and strengthening personal power.

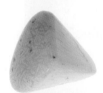

Scolecite sets life energy flowing unobtrusively and helps with gathering energy, which is expressed by fitness, productivity, and less need for sleep.

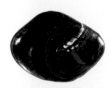

Tiger iron mobilizes reserves (the "tiger in the tank"). Works with enormous speed against fatigue, exhaustion, and lack of energy; raises productivity and stamina.

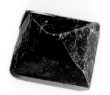

Zircon provides energy that remains within, helping to ensure survival and preventing tiredness and weakness from interfering with plans.

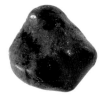

Zoisite (with ruby crystals) strengthens life energy, helps in recovering from severe deficiencies, and supports the rebuilding of energy reserves.

FERTILITY

Fertility and reproduction are at the basis of the kidney function area. The ability to conceive children is an expression of human vitality, and the intensity of the sex drive is directly connected with the condition of the kidneys' energy.

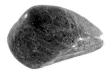

Epidote has a rebuilding and strengthening effect when sexual activity leads (occasionally or always) to persistent exhaustion and energy loss.

Hematite increases the vitality of the whole body, thus supporting an active sex life. Helpful for absence of menstruation caused by iron deficiency.

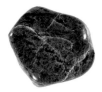

Nephrite promotes fertility and strengthens the function of the sex organs. Helpful for hormonal disturbances and sexual difficulty due to weakness or lack of energy.

Obsidian releases inhibitions and mobilizes life energy during sexual activity. Helpful for impotence and frigidity, and improves sexual performance.

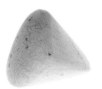

Scolecite promotes reproduction in both sexes by improving sperm production and fertility.

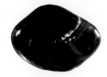

Tiger iron raises energy level and enhances sexual performance. Helpful for infertility due to general lack of energy, and for amenorrhea due to lack of iron.

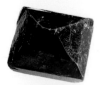

Zircon promotes fertility; helpful for disturbances in the menstrual cycle, especially late periods and very severe pain.

Zoisite (with ruby crystals) is helpful for afflictions of the testes and ovaries; promotes fertility; strengthens potency.

STRONG WILL AND POWER

The power and intensity of will are strongly dependent on the energy of the kidney function area. In traditional Chinese medicine, the ability to make compromises—with others and with oneself—is also part of the force of will. The aim here is to be as determined as water, taking all possible routes, always reaching its goal. This is shown by the ability to get past obstacles and distractions, or to include them in plans without being deterred from the goal itself. This is the ability to "do" and hence to gain power over one's own life.

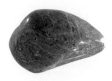

Epidote helps us to adapt easily to changing situations while still remaining true to our own goals, or even rediscovering them when they have been lost. Helps us to go our own way without straining.

Hematite strengthens the will and makes us aware of unfulfilled wishes in life. Improves the capacity to survive, and consequently the ability to improve living conditions.

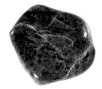

Nephrite helps us to find a balance between our own wishes and the demands of others, and yet to pursue our own path even in times of pressure and resistance.

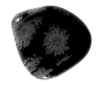

Obsidian helps us to deal with things that undermine our power and strength of will. Promotes self-mastery and defense against external attacks.

Scolecite strengthens cohesion in relationships and organizations; promotes team spirit, and therefore is helpful when goals can be reached only by group effort.

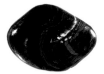

Tiger iron strengthens will and assertiveness; provides the energy and dynamism needed to master all obstacles.

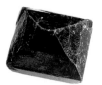

Zircon renders an unshakeable will and continual perseverance for reaching every goal that is truly important and meaningful in life.

Zoisite (with ruby crystals) strengthens the will and frees us from conformity and others' moods in order to realize our own ideas and wishes.

THE EARS AND HEARING

In traditional Chinese medicine, the kidneys are viewed as deep pools in which energy, power, and also memories are collected. The absorption of sounds also belongs to this collecting function. Sharpness of hearing is directly linked to the strength of the kidneys.

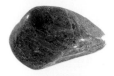

Epidote is helpful for hearing impairment when accompanied by a general weakness of the organism.

Hematite improves energy supply to the ears and strengthens the sense of hearing.

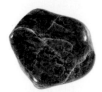

Nephrite is helpful for tinnitus (noise in the ears) under stress and pressure, or when present in connection with weak kidneys (and possibly liver blockage).

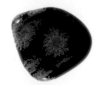

Obsidian is helpful for ear and hearing problems following traumatic events (for example, blast or gunfire trauma).

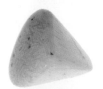

Scolecite sharpens the sense of hearing and helps in hearing the most subtle noises at great distances, as well as in distinguishing sounds and tones.

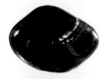

Tiger iron improves energy supply to the ears, strengthening the sense of hearing, especially when it is affected by fatigue.

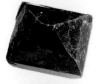

Zircon improves the sense of hearing by generally strengthening kidney energy.

Zoisite (with ruby crystals) helps with hearing impairment following hearing loss or ear disease, as well as general weakness.

MATURING AND AGING

The aging process is accompanied by the slow exhaustion of life energy—using up the jing energy we received at conception. When life energy is finally consumed, death follows. Aging, and the accompanying maturation brought about by the accumulation of experience, has its home in the kidney function area, just as conception does.

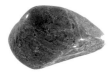 **Epidote** promotes spiritual maturity by banishing false self-images, keeping us spiritually young and vital even in old age.

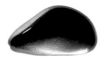 **Hematite** helps us to face life experiences and continually gain new energy through processing them.

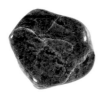 **Nephrite** promotes the maturation process, staying benevolent, tolerant, and "on top of things" as we get older but also preserving individual identity.

 Obsidian encourages jumping into life's experiences and coming through them unscathed, despite a few falls.

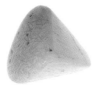 **Scolecite** enables us to accept aging and diminished energy, and to take pleasure in the positive aspects of every phase of life.

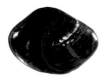 **Tiger iron** helps in accepting life's challenges and prospering from them. Brings maturity via the principle of "trial and error."

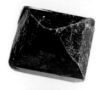

Zircon shows the transitory nature of all being, helps us free ourselves from restrictions, and leads us to the truly important things in life.

Zoisite (with ruby crystals) leads us to savor life to the fullest and use it constructively. Maintains youth and vitality well into old age.

DISTURBANCES IN THE KIDNEYS

When the kidneys function excessively, their energy is used up too quickly. This leads to phenomena such as restlessness, hectic behavior, sleeplessness, and a very strong, even excessive sex drive.

The physical symptoms are accompanied by an inclination to view one's own will as too important, leading one to impose it on others and in extreme cases, even to force it. Imperiousness and hunger for power are the consequences; here power does not mean "being able to do" but rather "forcing others to do," even (or precisely) when they do not want to. Here, the freedom to act according to one's own wishes turns into a compulsion to influence and control others.

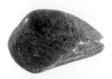

Epidote lends patience and makes it possible to find the right pace for activities. Helps eliminate self-importance and promotes quiet, healing sleep.

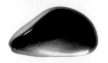

Hematite brings levelheadedness in actions and helps for arranging activities fittingly, so that using "brawn instead of brain" is only done when there is absolutely no way to avoid it.

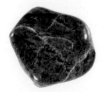

Nephrite has a balancing effect in hectic, restless times; helpful to quell an excessive sex drive and a desire for power and control.

Obsidian brings awareness of the dark side of false power and helps us admit our own mistakes and misdeeds, thus conquering them.

Scolecite stops energy depletion resulting from excessive activity, quells excessive sexual desire, and promotes good sleep.

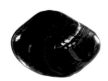

Tiger iron helps us to finish incomplete things, thus reducing energy loss in the kidneys. Also reduces desire for power, which in fact arises from the feeling of having too little control over one's own life.

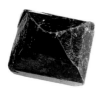

Zircon helps us deal with power levelheadedly, since "power is not eternal." Frees us from self-importance and destructive sexual impulses.

Zoisite (with ruby crystals) retains and rebuilds kidney energy, thus alleviating extreme situations. Helps avoid sexual performance anxiety and find the way back to a relaxed, natural sex life.

Weak kidney energy manifests in the form of a general lack of energy in life. This is connected with a weak will, listlessness, a feeling that one is a victim, and a life full of fear and anxiety.

Physically, fertility and sexual performance become hampered. A strong need for sleep and rest arises, and the affected person feels easily overstrained.

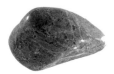

Epidote is helpful for severe lack of energy, listlessness, and a feeling of being continually stressed out. Gives energy and confidence, and helps with overcoming frustration.

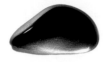

Hematite brings energy, strength, and a feeling of mastering life with one's own power. Awakens the "inner warrior," banishing any feelings of being a victim.

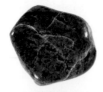

Nephrite gathers inner energy to conquer listlessness and excessive need for rest. Alleviates fear and anxiety and supports a stable inner balance.

Obsidian helps us sense our own power and force without being afraid of it. Strengthens the will, gives energy, and alleviates fear and feelings of being victimized.

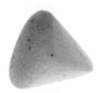

Scolecite regenerates exhausted kidney energy gently but continually. Leads us by degrees out of self-pity, lack of will, and listlessness. Helps us to view and accept life positively.

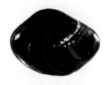

Tiger iron strengthens the will and drive, mobilizes energy reserves, and ensures that these will be refilled. Quickly returns the feeling of having a grip on life.

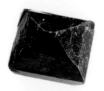

Zircon helps us overcome fear, anxiety, and victimization, and face life calmly in the knowledge that the necessary force will always be there when it's needed.

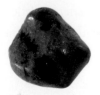

Zoisite (with ruby crystals) quickly regenerates completely exhausted energy. Pulls us out of deep exhaustion and brings swift healing.

STRENGTHENING THE KIDNEYS

To strengthen the kidneys, the same indications apply in principle as were given for the bladder. Drinking pure water and avoiding intoxicants (especially alcohol, caffeine, and strong medication) is particularly important. The kidneys are especially weakened by anxiety and shock, so it is expressly advised to treat and resolve these conditions with the appropriate means.

The energy of the kidneys can also be strengthened by a fulfilling, but not excessive, sex life.

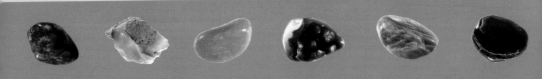

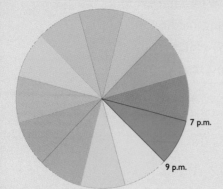

7 p.m.

9 p.m.

The Pericardium
(Sexual System)

ACCORDING TO THE ORGAN CLOCK, now is the ideal time for sex. However, not many people use this time for that purpose, except perhaps those who start the day at 3:00 every morning. But because monks—the only people usually up at that hour—traditionally have little opportunity to enjoy their sexuality, this population is even smaller. For most people, this is simply the time when the day's work is over and they can finally rest.

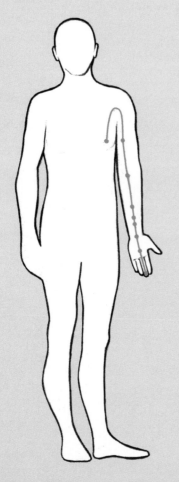

Pericardium meridian

124

PROTECTING THE HEART

The pericardium function area, sometimes called the heart circuit or circuit of sexuality, mainly serves to protect the heart by taking over a portion of its duties. For the Chinese, the heart is the seat of the spirit; thus it is what makes a person's true personality, or true being. In such a prominent position, it is especially vulnerable to attack, disturbance, and influence from outside. Because it is the task of the heart to open itself and to make connections, it is difficult for it to protect itself from harmful influences. This task is taken over by the pericardium function area, which defends the heart from all damaging influences (both physical and psychic). Psychic attacks, such as intentional or unintentional hurt and disappointment, always hit the pericardium function area first. Only when this area is truly weakened will the heart itself be affected and drawn in.

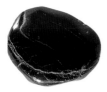

Almandine garnet releases the strength to master one's own life during crises and hard times. Strengthens resistance against negative influences of this kind.

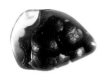

Fire agate promotes a positive, confident, and predominantly happy worldview, and also bestows the power to resist harmful influences.

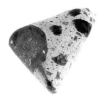

Fire opal brings enthusiasm into life, encouraging realization of true spiritual purpose. Helps us to simply shrug off attacks and disturbances.

Heliotrope is very important for supporting the pericardium. It gives the discretion to self-limit and maintain control over life, and also helps prevent physical damage to the heart (for example, heart attacks).

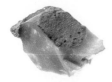

Precious opal conveys a joyful attitude toward earthly life and strengthens the will to live. This attitude toward life protects against harmful influences, or at least reduces their effects.

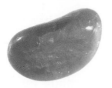

Rhodochrosite promotes a positive, enthusiastic attitude in life, and stimulates undiscriminating, all-embracing love. This attitude toward life is the best protection against attack, injury, and disappointment.

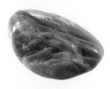

Sunstone affirms life and optimism, letting strengths shine forth. Lends energy for dealing with, and overcoming, negative influences and their consequences.

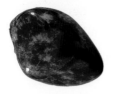

Thulite brings joy of life to all levels, stimulating life energy. Helps in confronting obstacles and challenges, making them downright inspirational.

RELAXATION AND ENJOYMENT

The task of the pericardium function area is to connect the pleasures of the ruler (the heart) with those of the subjects (the other function areas). The pericardium is responsible for relaxation and for the ability to let work be work and enjoy what life has to offer. Someone with a healthy pericardium can call it a day, clock out, and enjoy life without neglecting life's demands.

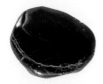

Almandine garnet increases joy and confidence in life, even when conditions are anything but pleasant and comfortable.

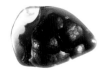

Fire agate supports disconnecting from work and responsibilities, drawing new energy from relaxation and enjoyable activities.

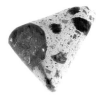

Fire opal inspires us to throw ourselves completely into the pleasures and joys of life and to give free rein to the enjoyment of living.

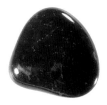

Heliotrope reveals serenity and inner peace even in times of stress and worry, instilling the confidence to accept and grapple with anything that happens.

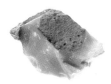

Precious opal reveals the many beautiful and colorful sides of life, and supports enjoying them to the fullest. Encourages staying completely present in the here and now.

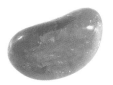

Rhodochrosite helps us to be joyful and unprejudiced, and to go about life playfully. Ensures that pleasure and enjoyment will not pass too quickly.

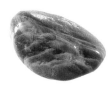

Sunstone propels us swiftly out of troubled times and gloomy states of mind into a joyful, cheery mood, rejoicing in existence.

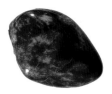

Thulite inspires happiness and pleasure in many facets of existence: in beauty, adventure, melancholy, romance, even in unnerving and bizarre experiences.

PLEASURE AND EROTICISM

Eroticism, one of the most enjoyable experiences, naturally belongs to the domain of pleasure, which is within the pericardium function area. Whereas the function area of the kidneys governs the aspect of reproduction, the area of the pericardium rules the pleasure and gratification associated with it. In everything from the fun of flirting to a joyful night of extensive lovemaking, erotic intensity is dependent on the energy of this function area.

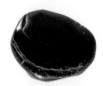

Almandine garnet overcomes unnecessary inhibitions and taboos, bringing pleasure in well-balanced sexuality (avoiding extremes).

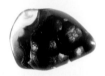

Fire agate connects enjoyment of sexuality with warmheartedness and faithfulness, promoting an atmosphere of comforting security.

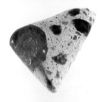

Fire opal awakens the inner fire and makes sex more fun. Makes us impulsive, lively, open-minded, willing to take risks, and therefore ready for some thrills.

Heliotrope protects sexual boundaries and instills respect for a partner's boundaries.

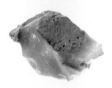

Precious opal strengthens desire, eroticism, and sexuality. Makes us alluring, unconventional, and fun-loving, always ready for new adventures.

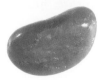

Rhodochrosite brings the erotic spark into flirting; brings liveliness, intensity, and fun to sexuality, and allows for the fullest pleasure in lovemaking.

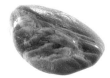 **Sunstone** promotes self-confidence in sexuality; helps us to stand by our own needs and wishes, and to communicate and fulfill them.

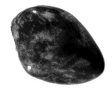 **Thulite** inspires enjoyment of lust, desire, sensuality, and sexuality to the fullest, throwing aside inhibitions and completely submerging in erotic pleasure.

THE LIGHTNESS OF BEING

A strong, well-balanced pericardium function area is revealed by ease in living and joy at being alive. Pleasure and enjoyment play a significant role in all activities.

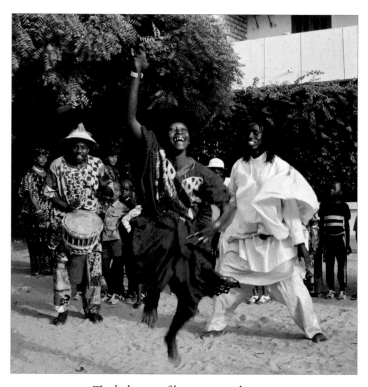

The lightness of being—joie de vivre

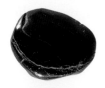

Almandine garnet helps in getting through very difficult times more easily, and in approaching even challenging and uncomfortable things happily.

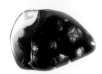

Fire agate integrates pleasure and enjoyment into the working world, and a joyful inner contentment into all areas of life.

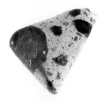

Fire opal awakens and animates, making us dynamic, lively, open-minded, and always ready for new things. Stimulates mischievous playfulness and makes life more fun.

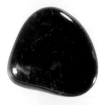

Heliotrope helps define limits, thus preserving a free space without pressure and negative influences, in which to remain lighthearted and relaxed.

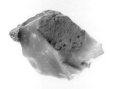

Precious opal makes us easygoing and brings lightness to being in the form of a colorful, glittering, many-faceted life full of variety and diversion.

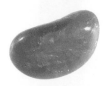

Rhodochrosite lightens the heart so that work is done effortlessly. Feelings are expressed spontaneously, and life acquires a certain nonchalance.

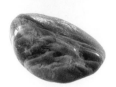

Sunstone leads us to the positive side of life and self, trusting optimistically and joyfully that there will be happiness in life.

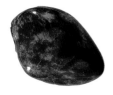

Thulite provides zest for all the aspects and shades of life, so it can be viewed as a fascinating, thrilling, exciting game.

DISTURBANCES IN THE PERICARDIUM

Excessive pericardium function mostly causes overexcitability but can also manifest as an inability to concentrate for long periods and as absentmindedness. People with such an imbalance may become fixated upon pleasures and diversions, momentary enjoyment being more important for them than long-term consequences. This is especially true in the sexual domain, where they will have a strong inclination to take advantage of every opportunity, even if it means putting a relationship of many years in jeopardy. They often are unable to bear difficult situations or to deal with criticism of their personality.

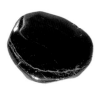

Almandine garnet promotes concentration, stamina, and self-control. Helps dispel obsessions with distractions and pleasure, and to endure uncomfortable situations.

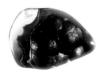

Fire agate supports being more reliable in times of absentmindedness and distraction; promotes awareness of responsibility, and maintaining a lasting interest in things.

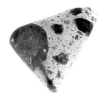

Fire opal helps avoid taking life too seriously, becoming more casual, and bearing uncomfortable situations with greater fortitude.

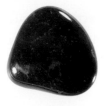

Heliotrope helps with disturbances in concentration, insomnia, and excessive excitability. Shows consequences of actions and supports acceptance of criticism.

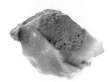

Precious opal calms and reminds us not to be too self-important. By way of a sincere, deeply felt joy in life, enables release of fixations on superficial pleasures.

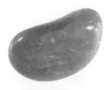

Rhodochrosite stimulates our attention, thus enabling protracted concentration when there is true interest.

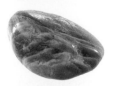

Sunstone promotes awareness of responsibility, dispels obsession with pleasure and distractions, and helps us to gather and focus attention.

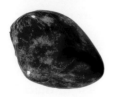

Thulite calms excessive excitability so we can face all of life with relish, yet place the importance of individual pleasures in perspective.

Suppressed pericardium function leads, in extreme cases, to a complete lack of liveliness and enjoyment of life. It often manifests as chronic nervousness and absentmindedness, as well as the inability to take pleasure in living. Even when there is an opportunity for relaxation and enjoyment, the affected person will still find reasons not to seize it. Often, such a person cannot have a playful sex life but simply satisfies sexual urges very quickly.

Both types of imbalance in the pericardium often lead to problems sleeping, frequently connected with intense dreams.

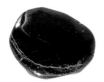

Almandine garnet brings alertness; helps with nervousness; and gives courage, hope, and confidence, imparting a fundamentally positive attitude toward life.

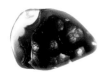

Fire agate is helpful for nervousness and absent-mindedness; encourages relaxation and is very effective for restless, frequently interrupted sleep.

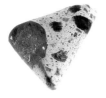

Fire opal awakens the "animal spirit," promotes the ability to enjoy things, and helps in discovering and experiencing the fun, happy aspects of sexuality.

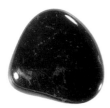

Heliotrope calms chronic nervousness and helps internal composure. Enables taking advantage of little "islands" of relaxation in everyday life, and sleeping well.

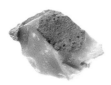

Precious opal confers liveliness, zest, and the joy of life. Helps with approaching life in a relaxed manner, and promotes good sleep.

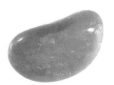

Rhodochrosite counteracts even a complete lack of liveliness and enjoyment. It has a swift, mood-lightening effect, stimulates enjoyment, and makes us awake and alert.

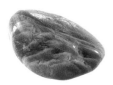

Sunstone brings joy, optimism, and zest for action. Also helpful for relaxation and alleviating nervousness. Allows healthy, worry-free sleep.

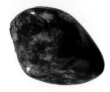 **Thulite** encourages enjoying life to the fullest, experiencing and enjoying sexuality, and finding pleasure in many areas of life. Also improves sleep.

STRENGTHENING THE PERICARDIUM

To strengthen the pericardium, all that is necessary is to set aside an adequate, but not excessive, place for relaxation and eroticism. Massage, dining out, saunas, a good vacation, and flirting for fun without any deep intent are all things that improve and strengthen the pericardium function area—as long as they are not practiced to excess or out of compulsion.

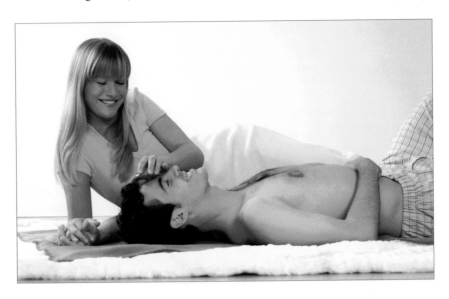

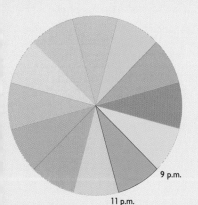

9 p.m.

11 p.m.

The Triple Heater

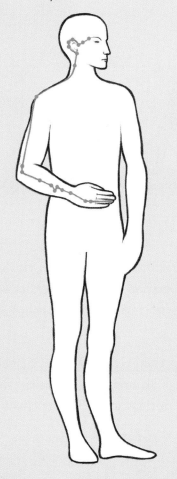

FROM THE POINT OF VIEW OF the organ clock, it is now time to rest. The body begins its nightly work of regeneration, which is best done without our interference. This regeneration begins with the optimization of the heat balance, which is one of the tasks of the triple heater.

Triple heater meridian

THE THREE HOT SPOTS

In the view of Chinese medicine, there are three "hot spots" inside the human body: the three Chou. These are the "lower heater," the "middle heater," and the "upper heater." The lower heater (the energy of the kidneys) represents a fire, which fuels a kettle (the digestive system), from which moisture rises. Consequently, the triple heater corresponds to breathing, digestion, and elimination.

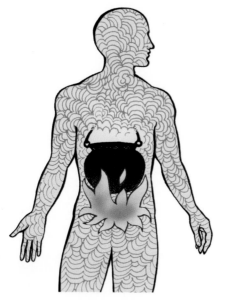

The three Chou—the body's hot spots

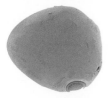

Carnelian stimulates increased energy in all three areas (breathing, digestion, elimination), thus having an invigorating effect on the entire organism.

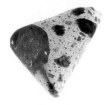

Fire opal stimulates energy generation in the body. It's often perceived as invigorating rather than warming but has a distinct strengthening effect on the triple heater.

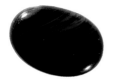

Mahogany obsidian enhances the burning process in the organism, thus raising the energy level. Has a perceptible warming effect.

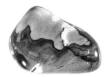

Mookaite (red) improves energy absorption from food and promotes comfortable warmth throughout the whole body.

Pyrope garnet makes energy generation in the body resistant to cold, weakness, fatigue, and other stress factors.

Red jasper enhances energy production, especially in times of need. When required, it raises body temperature to create fever, one of the body's greatest self-healing mechanisms.

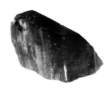

Red tourmaline stimulates not so much the generation of energy but rather its distribution. Efficient distribution means that less energy as a whole is required.

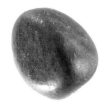

Ruby stimulates energy generation in the body and causes it to be applied optimally to specific needs. Helps prevent exhaustion from "excessive burning."

THE HUMAN HEATING SYSTEM

The triple heater does not exist as an organ structure. It essentially describes the manner in which body heat is produced, distributed, and used. A strong, well-balanced triple heater ensures that at any given time, enough energy will be produced and distributed, warming every part of the body appropriately. Psychic warmth, and the ability to give and receive a feeling of security, also depend on the condition of the triple heater—as well as the spleen and stomach function areas.

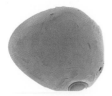

Carnelian improves energy balance between under-supplied, cool regions and regions with an energy surplus. Helps us not only to perceive psychic warmth but also to impart it.

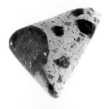

Fire opal improves distribution of energy in the body and inspires radiating warmth of heart evenly throughout all aspects of life.

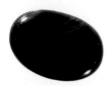

Mahogany obsidian promotes swift warming throughout the entire body; warms chronically cold hands and feet. Leads to rediscovering the lost sense of security.

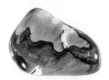

Mookaite (red) helps resolve energy imbalance and promotes radiation of friendly warmth between people.

Pyrope garnet brings about a constant warming of the entire body, and helps to maintain and radiate inner psychic warmth, even in times of crisis.

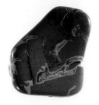

Red jasper brings about an even warming of the whole body, and supplies energy to make others feel secure, even in difficult situations.

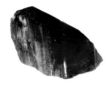 **Red tourmaline** brings about a gentle distribution of energy throughout the body, barely perceptible as warmth. This is clearly expressed as psychic warmth in the form of generosity and charm.

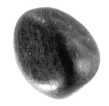 **Ruby** stabilizes energy generation in the body to a level that makes broad energy distribution possible. Makes us upbeat, friendly, and ready to help.

STRENGTHENING IMMUNITY

A side effect of the ability to supply each area of the body with an appropriate measure of energy and warmth is the maintenance of the body's defenses. Someone who is not freezing and has all the energy that is needed will not get sick. A strong and balanced triple heater will always convey the energy of the kidneys—the basis of immunity— at the right time to where it is needed, thus preventing weakness and illness.

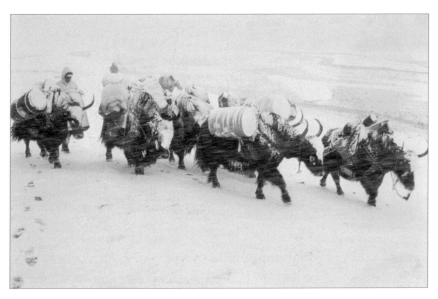

Resilience: the expression of a strong triple heater

Carnelian strengthens resilience by stimulating energy production and good energy distribution. Especially good for flu, colds, and similar ailments accompanied by fever.

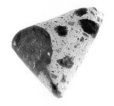

Fire opal maintains health with a good energy level and flexible distribution of energy. Very helpful for illness resulting from general lack of energy; also reduces fever.

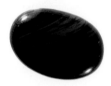

Mahogany obsidian strongly increases energy production; should only be used preventively in cases of weakness, sensation of cold, and other indicators of energy deficiency. Often too "hot" for acute illnesses, and therefore to be avoided.

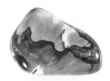

Mookaite (red) promotes a stable, quickly reacting immune system through efficient energy production and well-balanced distribution.

Pyrope garnet strengthens the body's defenses by means of stable energy production and distribution, even in cases of infection and inflammation.

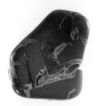

Red jasper strengthens immunity by raising the energy level. If needed, reduces fever during illness.

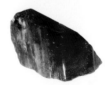

Red tourmaline keeps the body's defenses in motion by improving energy distribution. Therefore supports health when little energy is available due to weakness or exhaustion.

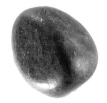

Ruby strengthens immunity in cases of a complete lack of energy (weakness, exhaustion) by strongly stimulating energy production. Has a strong fever-reducing effect, especially when the fever was initially necessary but then lingers.

DISTURBANCES IN THE TRIPLE HEATER

Excessive triple heater function imposes too much control on the coordination of body heat (the three Chou); the inner fires cannot burn freely, and lightheartedness and enjoyment of life are lost. Physically, this means the required warmth is not supplied to the necessary degree, which leads to an incorrect level of body heat. This takes the form either of too much heat or not enough (in both cases affecting the whole body), pervasive and independent of the external temperature.

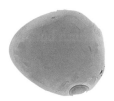

Carnelian offers impetus and good moods; has an enlivening and warming effect. Helps when insufficient body heat leads to shivering, weakness, or a disposition to illness.

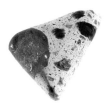

Fire opal brings easiness and joy to living, allowing us not to take life too seriously. Has a regulating effect on weaknesses in the body due to heat and cold.

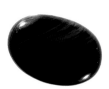

Mahogany obsidian releases excessive control over the coordination of warmth, often resulting in an immediate surge of heat followed by a well-balanced regulation of warmth. Psychically, often produces a surge of activity followed by relaxed joy at being alive.

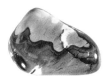

Mookaite (red) brings vitality and happiness. Helps balance out both lack of warmth and excessive heat.

Pyrope garnet maintains enjoyment of life even in difficult situations and balances out both lack of energy and excessive heat.

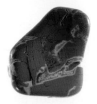

Red jasper fans the inner fire when it is not burning enough; therefore helps with a physical lack of warmth as well as psychically with listlessness, dejection, and lapsed interest in life.

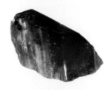

Red tourmaline makes us lighthearted and relaxed; promotes an appropriate coordination of warmth, adapted to the situation. Regulates both lack of warmth and excessive heat.

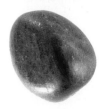

Ruby stokes the inner fire when it threatens to go out. Mostly helpful for insufficient warmth but also helps to curb excessive heat.

A suppressed triple heater function means that the three Chou are not connecting properly with one another. Some parts of the body are overheated while others are ice cold, causing mayhem from hot flushes and chills, sometimes simultaneously. This weakness in coordination manifests as sensitivity to any change in the weather and an inclination to sickness. In the psychic domain the lack of coordination leads to chaotic and confused emotions, inner struggles, and constant fluctuation, as well as a tendency to withdraw inward.

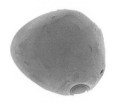

Carnelian calms the chaos of hot flushes and chills, and improves adaptability to weather changes. Also makes us more outgoing.

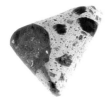

Fire opal leads to balanced distribution of warmth; reduces temperature sensitivity and general disposal toward sickness. Helps expansion following a period of withdrawal.

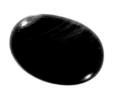

Mahogany obsidian is helpful for intense sensitivity to cold and in cases where shock or pain have muddled the triple heater. Dispels shock (even on the cellular level) and sets the self-regulation of heat in motion. Also calms the jumble of emotions in such situations.

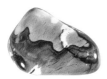

Mookaite (red) brings emotional balance and restores balance between turning inward and opening outward. Harmonizes the distribution of warmth and the perception of temperature.

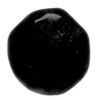

Pyrope garnet restores order to the coordination of warmth, and clears up chaotic and tumultuous feelings. Makes us impervious to changes in the weather.

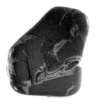

Red jasper stabilizes the coordination of warmth in the body and puts an end to psychic oscillation. Helps with coming out of a "shell" and overcoming inclination toward illness.

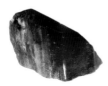

Red tourmaline clears up emotional chaos; harmonizes and stabilizes feelings. Immediately balances out chaotic coordination of warmth and calms extreme temperature sensations.

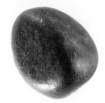

Ruby strengthens resistance to weather changes and illness; brings more emotional stability and extroversion. Improves coordination of warmth and regulates energy distribution.

STRENGTHENING THE TRIPLE HEATER

To strengthen the triple heater, it is especially helpful to have a regular sleep schedule and go to bed before 11:00 p.m., so that the body can have sufficient time for regeneration. One should also always wear clothes appropriate for the current temperature and avoid extreme temperatures if possible, including sunbathing.

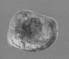

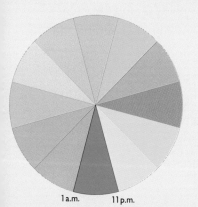

1 a.m.   11 p.m.

The Gallbladder

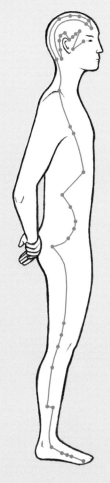

THE TIME OF THE GALLBLADDER should unequivocally be a time for sleep and regeneration. The gallbladder—and its partner function area, the liver—recuperates best while one is lying down, with as little disturbance from the mind as possible.

Gallbladder meridian

DECISIONS AND GROWTH

The gallbladder function area governs the ability to make decisions. The change phase of wood, to which the gallbladder and liver correspond, is responsible for growth and progress. The decisions made by the gallbladder function area relate to the body's growth and the development of the personality. The gallbladder's decision processes take place mostly subconsciously. Decisions about actual goals in life and how to reach them are, as a rule, not a function of the conscious intellect. Consequently it is best to let the gallbladder work during sleep and to wake up with a new decision the next morning, full of the energy needed to put it into action.

Aventurine strengthens resolution and individuality, makes it clear what causes joy and unhappiness, and what encourages making dreams come true.

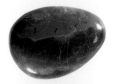

Chrysocolla strengthens the ability to adapt plans to changing situations and to make the right decisions.

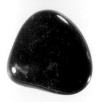

Heliotrope helps with quick adjustment to unforeseen situations and remaining in control in all areas.

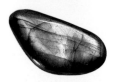

Labradorite works as an "illusion killer," giving a realistic evaluation of present conditions, thus laying the foundation for correct, lasting decisions.

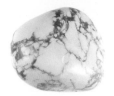

Magnesite brings patience and relaxation; promotes a life-affirming attitude. Helps defray pressure when making decisions, allowing free choice.

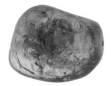

Peridot provides strength for making decisions, blocking out others' opinions and other outside influences.

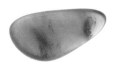

Serpentine (clinochrysotile) balances mood fluctuations and relieves inner tension, making it possible to find peaceful solutions for conflicts.

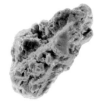

Turquoise helps us find inner peace and stop feeling like victims of circumstances. Strengthens the ability to recognize what the consequences of actions will be before the fact.

DETERMINATION AND COURAGE

Decisions of this kind require creativity, courage, and determination. A strong and balanced gallbladder function area enables clear decisions, commitment to new ideas and projects, exploration of new paths, and realization of goals that no one has achieved previously. A person with strong gallbladder energy tends to break past old conventions ("We've always done it that way") and blaze new trails.

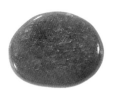

Aventurine, as the name may suggest (Italian *a ventura*, or by chance), helps in opening up to new things and developing complex ideas.

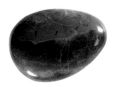

Chrysocolla supports consistently following a chosen path, even when it may seem anything but straightforward. Strengthens creativity and determination, and enables viewing life as a game in which beauty and justice lead to fulfillment.

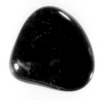 **Heliotrope** helps to develop what is truly important in life, and to protect it by combating bothersome influences with courage and determination.

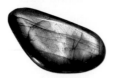 **Labradorite** stimulates courage and creativity, breaking past the boundaries of old rules and customs, and forging new paths.

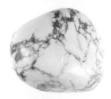 **Magnesite** relaxes our approach to life, helping us to bear hardships and pressures patiently, progressing steadily but without a struggle.

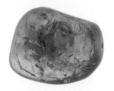 **Peridot** supports living life according to personal beliefs and not being manipulated by insinuation, reproach, or guilt.

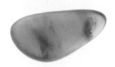 **Serpentine** (clinochrysotile) unifies an ability to compromise with a knack for preserving personal ideas and opinions and remaining true to personal goals.

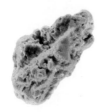 **Turquoise** enlivens and brings joy in activity. Instills awareness of being an artisan of personal happiness; strengthens steady progress along one's individual path.

EXPANDING AND GROWING

Going our own way and reaching our goals engenders a feeling of expansion. When we are able to do what we want, we are able to create our own space, and, ultimately, to live life freely according to our own

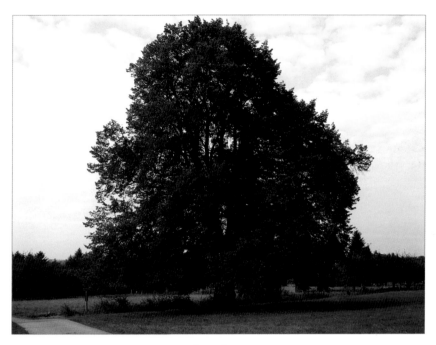

Growth and expansion

ideas. By realizing our plans, we grow both inwardly and outwardly, filling our place in the world and finding contentment.

Aventurine impalpably but steadily helps us expand our space and consequently to grow and develop in it, without self-restriction.

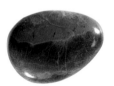

Chrysocolla strengthens growth and expansion; supports unrestricted development and living life in freedom and beauty.

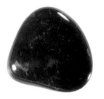

Heliotrope helps define and protect the space needed to grow and flourish, allowing for undisturbed development.

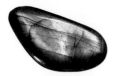

Labradorite, through spontaneous realizations, brings sudden expansion of the psychic space, resulting in developmental leaps forward.

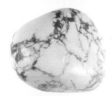

Magnesite helps expand our space through relaxation and calmness, which also support growth and development.

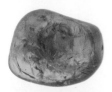

Peridot helps in creation of free space for growth, consciously and actively discarding all that is not truly owned.

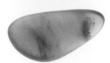

Serpentine (clinochrysotile) protects valuable free space and inner peace, on the basis of which harmoniously balanced development becomes possible.

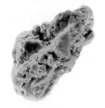

Turquoise helps stave off repressive influences that slow development. Fosters growth, expansion, and self-actualization.

IDEAS AND MOTIVATION

A strong gallbladder—along with a well-balanced liver function area—is expressed by a life full of ideas and motivation. Someone in whom these function areas are strong, besides being full of new ideas, also has the ability to pursue the goals arising from them steadily and persistently. It is easy to arouse such a person's enthusiasm, but only rarely will there be deviation from personal goals.

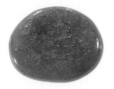

Aventurine brings a plethora of ideas and inspiration; also promotes tolerance and acceptance toward unfamiliar ideas and helps in choosing the "right" one and gradually implementing it at the proper pace without pressure or force.

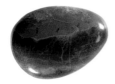

Chrysocolla brings great creativity and inspires not just the achievement of ideas "somehow," but also their beautification and refinement.

Heliotrope stimulates creative dreaming and helps for adhering to goals and avoiding distractions. Also enables retaining ideas until the right moment comes to step swiftly and directly into action.

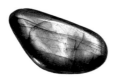

Labradorite promotes childlike enthusiasm, fantasy, and a wealth of ideas; also helps for choosing among these (not analytically, but through spontaneous perception) and implementing them.

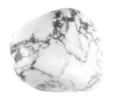

Magnesite makes it clear which ideas are truly important and supports allowing many of them to "just happen," by recognizing and nurturing favorable conditions.

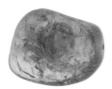

Peridot reinforces personal ideas in the face of resistance and, if necessary, supports fighting back in order to realize them.

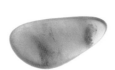

Serpentine (clinochrysotile) opens us to the ideas of others; also helps us to limit our own ideas, only espousing those that resonate. Brings steadfastness in the achievement of goals, but without pressure or stress.

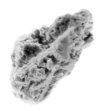

Turquoise helps in developing ideas, at first mentally until they are completely mature, then by stepping promptly and firmly into action.

DISTURBANCES
IN THE GALLBLADDER

Excessive gallbladder function occurs when decisions must be made under pressure or when goals cannot be realized due to external conditions. In these cases, freedom to act is restricted, leading to frustration and finally anger. Chronic excessive gallbladder function manifests in a tendency to overreact and have fits of rage. Physically, excessive gallbladder function is accompanied by chronic tension and hectic activity. Decisions are made too quickly, and it becomes more important to "do something" than to take the time to see that the right thing is done.

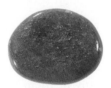

Aventurine helps to relieve inner pressure resulting from decision processes; instills patience, calms anger, and helps with tension. Calms inner unrest and promotes good sleep.

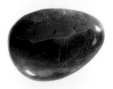

Chrysocolla helps to maintain a cool head and not be overcome by aggression. Encourages balance and control, and resolves frustration. Relieves tension and cramps.

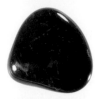

Heliotrope soothes irritation, aggression, and impatience. Helps in making decisions calmly and collectedly, even under pressure, and in preserving the ability to take action.

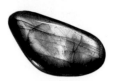

Labradorite assists recognition of decisions made too quickly or mistakenly. Cools hot-tempered reactions; supports returning to original ideas and realizing them.

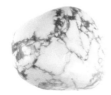

Magnesite soothes nervousness, irritation, and hectic activity; adds resilience, alleviates pressure in decision making, and supports patience during implementation of decisions. Generally relaxes and releases cramps.

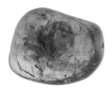

Peridot causes us to "unload" stored-up anger and bottled-up vexation, but promotes a constructive attitude after the cleansing storm. Makes it easier to admit mistakes and forgive them in others.

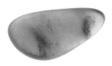

Serpentine (clinochrysotile) protects from hasty decision making, balances out mood fluctuations, and restores equilibrium and inner peace. Alleviates tension and the inclination toward aggressive behavior.

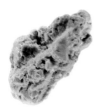

Turquoise restores the capacity to act and brings inner calm at times when frustration and resignation have changed into rage and aggression. Helpful for chronic tension and cramps.

Suppression in the gallbladder function area results in the inability to make decisions. This manifests as cowardice, a tendency to make excuses, or the complete denial of any responsibility. These weaknesses are often concealed by idleness, or by simply doing nothing until the problem has solved itself. Physically, deficient gallbladder function appears as a lack of resilience in the muscles and tendons, giving an overall impression of flabbiness.

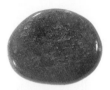

Aventurine inspires spontaneity, decisiveness, and enthusiasm; helpful for flabbiness and complaints of the muscles and tendons.

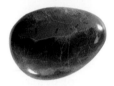

Chrysocolla is helpful for great decision difficulties; instills acceptance of changing situations and adhering to a chosen path despite ups and downs. Strengthens and reinforces muscles and tendons.

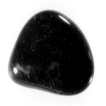

Heliotrope dispels hesitation and dithering; urges taking responsibility and overcoming weakness and idleness. Restores the capacity to act, also strengthening the tone and responsiveness of muscles and tendons.

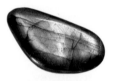

Labradorite helps in recognizing excuses for what they are (disintegrating them right in front of our eyes) and in taking responsibility.

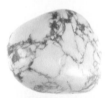

Magnesite helps in making levelheaded, determined decisions. Promotes resilience, tone, and flexibility in muscles and tendons.

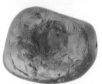

Peridot fosters decision making and risk taking, brings awareness of shortcomings, and encourages taking responsibility and, therefore, righting wrongs. Improves muscle responsiveness.

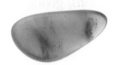

Serpentine (clinochrysotile) sustains in the face of difficult decisions, especially when cowardice has led to conflicts (and it becomes obvious that "sitting things out" is not sufficient to resolve them). Also strengthens muscles and tendons.

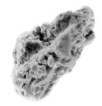

Turquoise supports taking responsibility in life and destiny. Increases muscle power and helps to overcome weakness.

STRENGTHENING THE GALLBLADDER

The weakest time of the gallbladder is between 11:00 a.m. and 1:00 p.m., twelve hours from its strongest time, as is the case with all function areas. To strengthen the gallbladder function area, it is very beneficial to take a nap, or at least a rest, during this time. Going to bed before 11:00 p.m. allows the gallbladder to work in peace during the night.

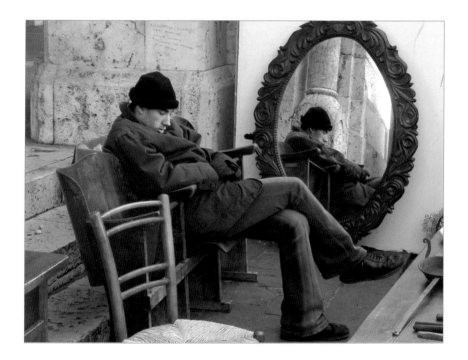

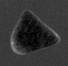 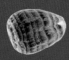 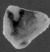 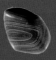 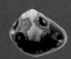

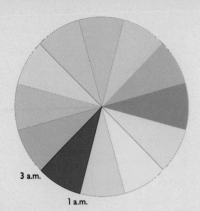

3 a.m.

1 a.m.

The Liver

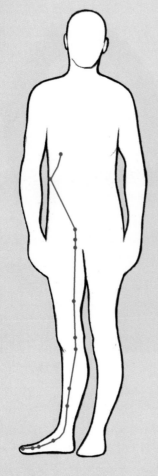

LIKE THE GALLBLADDER, THE LIVER works best during the night. It is best able to do its work when the conscious intellect is not interfering, so it is important to spend this time in sleep as often as possible.

Liver meridian

156

INNER PLANNING

The liver function area is responsible for planning. The flow of energy that is necessary for the operation of each function area is planned out and held in harmony by the liver. The liver sends chi (life energy) and blood in all directions and ensures the regularity that is necessary to maintain all the body's functions.

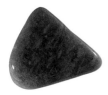 **Amazonite** inspires taking life's planning in hand, and provides free-flowing life energy. Brings a "magic touch" to all undertakings by way of a harmonic connection between intuition and understanding.

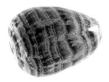 **Aragonite** promotes flexibility and tolerance in planning, and helps with staying concentrated on things if there is a tendency to be volatile. Promotes harmony throughout the organism.

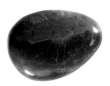 **Chrysocolla** inspires creative planning and allows plans to grow organically, one thing leading to the next, continuously being refined. Makes for a balanced combination of construction and decomposition within the organism.

 Chrysoprase improves aesthetic sense; helps us to see ourselves as a part of the whole and to adjust plans accordingly. In this way, our lives come into harmony with the natural order of things.

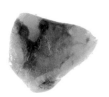 **Emerald** provides a deep understanding of personal life conditions and thus promotes planning that incorporates all the aspects of life harmoniously. Inspires living honorably and genuinely; and helps us to orient ourselves and find our way in times of crisis.

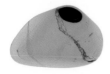 **Green fluorite** brings multifaceted ideas into a harmonious but still free order, allowing for changes and metamorphoses. This brings life and growth into balance.

 Malachite promotes a sense of beauty, friendship, sensuality, and justice, and orients life planning around these four pillars. Frees the flow of life energy and makes life intense and fulfilling.

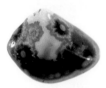 **Orbicular jasper** (ocean jasper) brings hope and confidence to life planning, and promotes a powerful stream of life, helping with implementation of plans.

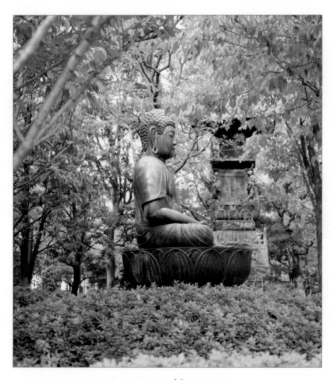

Serenity and harmony

INNER HARMONY

The equilibrium provided by the liver's planning brings harmony and relaxation to every part of the body. The liver function area harmonizes the emotions, releases tension, and promotes undisturbed well-being and harmony with the world surrounding us. It sets the body's energies in order and ensures that they will flow quietly and harmoniously. A well-balanced liver function area leads to a calm mood pervading the entire person.

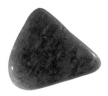

Amazonite calms agitated spirits and resolves conflict, antagonism, and feelings of inner dividedness. Eases disturbances in both psychic and physical growth.

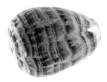

Aragonite promotes growth and harmonizes overly fast development that threatens to run off course. Helpful for inner unrest and nervous tremors.

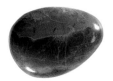

Chrysocolla helps bring individual plans into harmony with the surrounding world. Thus promotes harmony, inner equilibrium, and strong growth.

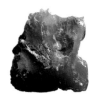

Chrysoprase strengthens trust in the harmony of the world, thereby enabling a harmonious life in accordance with natural conditions. Promotes psychic and bodily cleansing for the restoration or maintenance of inner harmony.

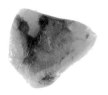

Emerald promotes purposeful spiritual growth as well as strong, harmonious physical well-being. Helps in overcoming blows from fate, makes us balanced and open, and improves our adjustment to surroundings.

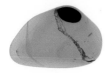

Green fluorite regulates excessive or deficient growth and ensures that a healthy equilibrium is preserved, along with the natural order of things.

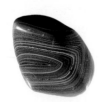

Malachite brings liveliness and intensity, releases inhibitions, encourages adventurousness and risk taking, and brings a healthy growth impulse. This force leads to a vital harmony of development and expansion, in which a great deal of energy can be guided and channeled.

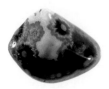

Orbicular jasper (ocean jasper) helps in resolving inner conflicts and achieving a positive view of life. From this grows stable harmony that can withstand pressure, making undisturbed growth possible and bringing all developments into unison.

A CLEAR VIEW

Good planning is connected with the ability to act with good foresight. To have good foresight, one must be able to see. The function area of the liver, therefore, opens through the eyes. The state of the eyes and sharpness of vision are directly linked to the condition of the liver. A harmonious liver makes a clear view possible and enables one to see what is really present.

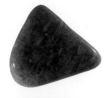

Amazonite helps us to be entirely present spiritually and to remain attentive and concentrated on matters. Also helps with disturbances in sight caused by the optic nerve.

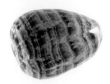

Aragonite frees fixations on specific beliefs that obscure vision. Physically, relaxes the area of the eyes.

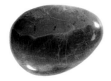

Chrysocolla promotes clarity and neutrality, and the ability to see things as they are, without judgment or bias. Helpful for eye infections.

Chrysoprase changes the "perception filter" with which people try to affirm their own ideas through selective perception, substituting a benign view of things. Also helpful for many eye afflictions.

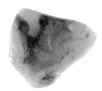

Emerald brings spiritual clarity, wakefulness, and farsightedness. One of the most important stones for the eyes. Helpful for tired eyes, eye infections, glaucoma, cataracts, myopia, farsightedness, weak vision, and optic nerve problems.

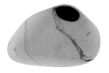

Green fluorite helps remedy fixed ideas, limitations, narrow-mindedness, insularity, and restrictive thought and behavior patterns, making a clear view of things possible. Helpful for weak eyes and failing eyesight.

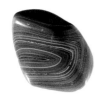

Malachite improves the gift for observation and enables information to be grasped more quickly, broadening the horizons of the imagination. Malachite also intensifies the physical sense of sight and sharpness of vision.

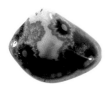

Orbicular jasper (ocean jasper) focuses our vision unwaveringly and hopefully into the future, enabling us to act with foresight. Helpful for all organic eye problems, from conjunctivitis to glaucoma.

MOVEMENT

The liver is responsible for an equitable distribution of the chi, as well as for the regularity of the body's movements. In order to be able to move and keep one's body straight, the muscles and tendons must be used. The ability to contract, just like the ability to relax, is part of the liver function area. The strength of a well-balanced liver function area can be seen in the consistent body control of athletes.

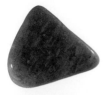

Amazonite improves spiritual and bodily movements, and helps with muscle and tendon problems such as carpal tunnel syndrome, tendinitis, or tennis elbow.

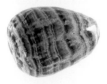

Aragonite makes us spiritually flexible and adaptable; harmonizes bodily movements. Strengthens muscles, tendons, slipped discs, and menisci (knee cartilage), and helps with complaints in these areas.

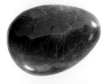

Chrysocolla brings elasticity and flexibility to body and spirit. Strengthens the musculature and loosens cramped tendons, thereby also helping with carpal tunnel syndrome, tendinitis, and tennis elbow.

Chrysoprase helps dispel psychic pressure and remove blockage in the body. Eliminates feelings of physical weight and heaviness, and improves movement.

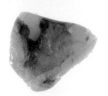

Emerald promotes both the ability to tense and the ability to relax. Improves coordination and engenders energetic, purposeful movement as well as good body control.

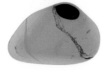

Green fluorite loosens rigid spirituality and fixed adherence to habits and trusted mechanisms. This leads to improved bodily movement.

Malachite promotes free movement and deep relaxation, which can turn at lightning speed to maximum tautness, then just as quickly back to relaxation—like a predatory animal. Makes reactions quick; strengthens muscles, tendons, and joints; and gives good body control.

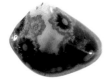

Orbicular jasper (ocean jasper) improves movement and the way the body feels; helps for recovering and regenerating quickly after exertion; relieves muscle aches and promotes the building of strong muscles and resilient tendons.

LIFE IN FLOW

When the liver's function is well balanced everything in life is fluent and in tune. Every task seems to complete itself, and demands grow in harmony with one's own capabilities.

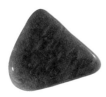

Amazonite helps in overcoming difficulties, hardships, and all hindering, restricting factors in life.

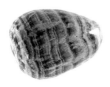

Aragonite brings life into a balanced flow, especially when overly rapid spiritual developments have led to mental overload or to dwindling interest in things.

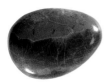

Chrysocolla offers strength of body, harmony of the soul, and mental acuity, making powerful spiritual development possible.

Chrysoprase increases confidence in life and the ability to embrace the flow of life. This enables overcoming even the most difficult challenges with comparative ease.

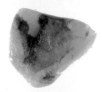

Emerald gives direction, power, and intensity, leading to a purposeful, successful life flow.

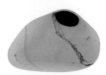

Green fluorite alleviates every form of spiritual and psychic rigidity, opening us to change and consequently bringing life (back) into the flow.

Malachite makes the flow of life into a powerful stream, full of new discoveries, challenges, and adventures; the resulting increased demands bring out the best in powers and capabilities.

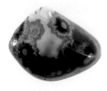

Orbicular jasper (ocean jasper) bestows life energy, a feeling of abundance, and awareness of limitless possibilities, abilities, and creativity. Brings life into flow, making possible a lasting improvement in life conditions.

DISTURBANCES IN THE LIVER

Excessive liver function causes life planning to falter and harmony to be lost. This leads to imbalance, stagnation, and blockages in both blood and emotions. The latter turn to aggression, which is bottled up until the gallbladder finally expresses it in the form of rage. Deep disturbances in the liver function area emerge physically as chronic muscle tension and halting, disjointed movements. In extreme cases, entire parts of the body can become wholly immovable.

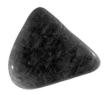

Amazonite has a balancing and calming effect on extreme mood fluctuations, relieves tension and cramps, and helps with stiffness and restricted movement.

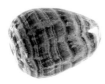

Aragonite is helpful for hypersensitivity, inner restlessness, and inconsistent, jerky, and uncontrolled movements.

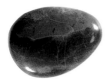

Chrysocolla helps us maintain a cool head when stressed, nervous, or overwrought. Softens expressed emotions and calms mood fluctuations. Helpful for severe muscle tension, cramps, and menstrual problems.

Chrysoprase helps to alleviate even the most intense feelings, such as jealousy and lovesickness; promotes trust and security in the self. Relieves stiffness and restricted movement resulting from poisoning.

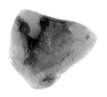

Emerald helps preserve clarity of thought and balanced emotions during crises and phases of disorientation. Promotes flexibility in the body and balanced muscle tone.

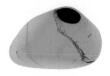

Green fluorite releases long-lasting tensions that have led to misshapen or shortened muscles and tendons. Also helpful for confused thoughts and suppressed feelings.

Malachite balances pent-up emotions or an excessive overflow of feelings (in either case this can lead to a cathartic outburst before inner peace is reached). Helps with cramps and menstrual problems, as well as stiffness and restricted movement caused by inflammation or illness (arthritis, rheumatism, gout).

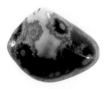

Orbicular jasper (ocean jasper) lends strength to tackle unresolved conflicts and releases pent-up aggression. Brings order to internal imbalances, both physical and psychic, and relieves chronic tension.

Suppressed liver function, on the other hand, manifests as weakness; because the ability to plan is too weak, the gallbladder cannot realize any plans either. This is expressed as constant dithering, often connected with difficulty in bringing one's life into order and keeping an eye on the big picture. Physically, this weakness of the liver shows itself in the form of weak or flabby muscles, loss of appetite, or poor eyesight.

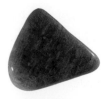

Amazonite is helpful for timidity and lack of capability. Banishes the idea of being a helpless victim of almighty fate.

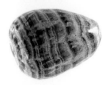

Aragonite helps with lack of energy and the feeling of being a failure in life. Improves appetite and strengthens musculature.

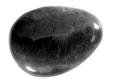

Chrysocolla gives new drive when we feel weak, sluggish, or dejected. Enlivens us and offers new vigor for taking on personal goals.

Chrysoprase helps create order in life, fundamentally removing all hindrances and inhibiting factors. Little by little, restores control over life's planning.

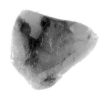

Emerald helps in overcoming weakness, promotes regeneration, and boosts energetic drive. Makes us motivated and purposeful; "opens our eyes" both spiritually and physically.

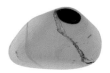

Green fluorite helps restore order in life and brings new ideas, rapid comprehension, and well-regulated energy.

Malachite brings fresh verve and momentum to life, pulling us out of lethargy and idleness. Speeds decision making so that it is spontaneous, without lengthy contemplation. This brings us (back) into motion and initiates a reorganization of life. Eases "spiritual birth" as well as physical childbirth.

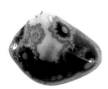

Orbicular jasper (ocean jasper) is helpful for exhaustion, enlivening in cases of chronic fatigue, brings good sleep, and promotes overall renewal and regeneration. Helps us to engage actively in shaping our lives.

STRENGTHENING THE LIVER

To strengthen the liver, relaxing activities are particularly important, in addition to getting sufficient sleep. Walks in the woods, exercises to improve motion (t'ai chi exercises are especially helpful in this regard), and meditation to ward off stress and tension all have a very strong balancing effect on the liver. A healthy diet with plenty of fresh food is also an important factor in ensuring the welfare of the liver function area.

Recommended Reading

Costelloe, Marina. *The Complete Guide to Crystal Astrology*. Findhorn, Scotland: Findhorn Press, 2007.

Fleck, Dagmar, and Liane Jochum. *Hot Stone and Gem Massage*. Rochester, Vt: Healing Arts Press, 2008.

Gienger, Michael. *Crystal Massage for Health and Healing*. Findhorn, Scotland: Findhorn Press, 2006.

———. *The Healing Crystal First Aid Manual*. Findhorn, Scotland: Findhorn Press, 2006.

———. Translated by Chinwendu Uzodike. *Healing Crystals: The A–Z Guide to 430 Gemstones*. Findhorn, Scotland: Findhorn Press, 2005.

———. *Purifying Crystals: How to Clear, Charge and Purify Your Healing Crystals*. Findhorn, Scotland: Findhorn Press, 2008.

Gienger, Michael, and Joachim Goebel. *Gem Water: How to Prepare and Use More Than 130 Crystal Waters for Therapeutic Treatments*. Findhorn, Scotland: Findhorn Press, 2008.

Grundmann, Monika. *Crystal Balance: A Step-by-Step Guide to Beauty and Health through Crystal Massage*. Findhorn, Scotland: Findhorn Press, 2008.

Guhr, Andreas, and Joerg Nagler. *Crystal Power: Mythology and History*. Findhorn, Scotland: Findhorn Press, 2006.

Silveira, Isabel. *Quartz Crystals*. Findhorn, Scotland: Findhorn Press, 2008.

Welch, Ricky. *Aurum Manus: The "Golden Hands" Method of Crystal-based Holistic Massage*. Findhorn, Scotland: Findhorn Press, 2006.

About the Authors

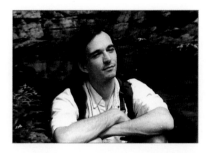

WOLFGANG MAIER

In 1989 Wolfgang Maier began a two-year shiatsu course that marked the beginning of his interest in traditional Chinese medicine (TCM). During his training in the use of healing stones with Michael Gienger and Cairn Elen, he decided to pursue his interest in the wisdom and fascinating observations of TCM. Because the concepts of TCM are often difficult for Westerners to grasp, he devoted himself for the next seven years to studying the fundamentals of TCM and expressing them in a simpler, more understandable form. He was the first to describe, in a logically comprehensible manner, TCM's many correspondences with the individual phases of change, based on the fundamental principles behind the phases. This made it possible to have a deeper understanding of TCM than can be achieved by simply memorizing the correspondences.

Fruitful collaboration with Michael Gienger then led to establishing the first hybrid of traditional Chinese medicine and the art of stone healing. Here TCM, with its millennia of acquired wisdom, takes on the role of a diagnostic system, while stone healing is applied in order to balance the disharmonies and energetic imbalances revealed in this process.

Wolfgang Maier has written the book *Der Mondschild* [The Moon Shield] (www.mondschild.de), which suggests an entirely new approach to the effects of lunar phases. Professionally, he works as an independent communications coach and problem solver, both in companies and privately. He holds lectures and seminars by request and offers something unavailable anywhere else in the world: a year-long course in traditional Chinese medicine and the art of healing stones. Further information on this can be found on the German website www.shk-tcm.de.

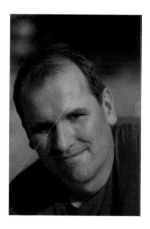

MICHAEL GIENGER

Michael Gienger has studied the organ clock since his shiatsu training in 1984 (shiatsu is the needle-free Japanese form of acupuncture) and stone healing since 1985. He has focused continuing efforts on linking the positive aspects of both systems, as summarized in *Die Organuhr* [The Organ Clock] (published in 1994, with Gerhard Kupka), and in his book *Heilsteine und Lebensrhythmen* [Healing Crystals and Life

Rhythms] (2001; earlier title: *Die Edelsteinuhr* [The Gem Clock]). The present book became possible after many years of intensive collaboration with Wolfgang Maier, starting in 1999. Michael Gienger contributed the descriptions of the effects of healing stones to this book. He has a unique ability to summarize the true essence of an astonishing body of knowledge.

As an internationally recognized expert, Michael Gienger has written many standard works on healing stones, including *Crystal Power, Crystal Healing; The Healing Crystal First Aid Manual; Healing Crystals: The A–Z Guide to 430 Gemstones; Crystal Massage for Health and Healing*; and *Gem Water: How to Prepare and Use More Than 130 Crystal Waters for Therapeutic Treatments*. His books have been translated into nine languages. Michael Gienger is cofounder of Steinheilkunde e. V. (1995), the Cairn Elen Lebensschule (1997), and the Cairn Elen Netzwerk (1998). Together with his wife, Anja, he oversees Cairn Elen editions at Neue Erde publishing. He also holds lectures and seminars on healing stones. More on Michael Gienger and his projects can be found on the following German websites:

> www.michael-gienger.de
> www.edelstein-massagen.de
> www.cairn-elen.de
> www.cairn-elen.net
> www.fairtrademinerals.de

Illustration Credits

Karin Attner: 169

Bruno Baumann (www.bruno-baumann.de): 139

Ines Blersch (www.inesblersch.de): Healing stone photos, plus 13, 18, 20, 22, 23, 129, 134, 170

Dragon Design: 10, 11, 17, 18, 21, 136

Myriam Höfer: 43

Atelier Bunter Hund: 32, 44, 55, 66, 77, 90, 100, 111, 124, 135, 145, 156

Wolfgang Maier: 6

www.photos.com: 57, 158

www.pixelio.de: i, ii–iii, 25, 33, 45, 50, 78, 91, 101, 105, 149, 155

Karola Sieber, red tourmaline photo used in the triple heater chapter

Ute Weigel: 113

Index

Page numbers in *italics* refer to images.

BOOKS OF RELATED INTEREST

Hot Stone and Gem Massage
by Dagmar Fleck and Liane Jochum

The Metaphysical Book of Gems and Crystals
by Florence Mégemont

Gemstone Reflexology
by Nora Kircher

The Healing Power of Gemstones
In Tantra, Ayurveda, and Astrology
by Harish Johari

Vibrational Medicine
The #1 Handbook of Subtle-Energy Therapies
by Richard Gerber, M.D.

The Handbook of Chinese Massage
Tui Na Techniques to Awaken Body and Mind
by Maria Mercati

Chinese Pediatric Massage
A Practitioner's Guide
by Kyle Cline, L.M.T.

Chinese Massage for Infants and Children
Traditional Techniques for Alleviating Colic, Colds, Earaches,
and Other Common Childhood Conditions
by Kyle Cline, L.M.T.

INNER TRADITIONS • BEAR & COMPANY
P.O. Box 388
Rochester, VT 05767
1-800-246-8648
www.InnerTraditions.com

Or contact your local bookseller